DIOXIN,
AGENT ORANGE
The Facts

Michael Gough

Plenum Press • New York and London

Library of Congress Cataloging in Publication Data

Gough, Michael, 1939–
  Dioxin, agent orange.

  Bibliography: p.
  Includes index.
  1. Dioxins—Toxicology. 2. Dioxins—Environmental aspects. I. Title.
RA1242.D55G68   1986   363.1'79   86-467
ISBN 0-306-42247-6

© 1986 Michael Gough

Plenum Press is a division of
Plenum Publishing Corporation
233 Spring Street, New York, N.Y. 10013

Printed in the United States of America

For Lee, Laura, and Barry

PREFACE

Dioxin lurks seemingly everywhere, as though spread around the country by some malevolent force. Undetectable to the human senses, dioxin has been found by use of sophisticated scientific apparatus in expected places, like old chemical plants and chemical dumps, and unexpected places, like people's front yards, pristine lakes in virgin forests, and Boy Scout encampments. Each discovery sets off a wave of headlines and controversies about human health. In newspapers and news programs, experts from universities and public interest groups highlight predictions of dire tragedies, bracketing the word "dioxin" with "cancer-causing chemical" and "most toxic chemical known." In the same article or newscast, experts from chemical companies and various levels of government generally respond with unsuccessful reassurances that the risks are exaggerated. In some cases, the soothing words are belied by the government's providing elaborate protective devices to the workers it sends to sample the same area where it had downplayed the risks. As days pass, the news value of the story declines, and the latest dioxin story fades away, perhaps to oblivion, perhaps to later resurrection as a reminder of the prevalence of the dioxin risk when yet another discovery is made. The story has no resolution; it just goes away.

What are people who are neither experts nor partisans in the struggles about environmental health to make of the conflicting interpretations, opinions, and actions? No one wants to be poisoned by an unseen, undetected toxic substance, and if the experts who warn of disaster are correct, decisive action must be taken to reduce the risks associated with dioxin in our environment. On the other hand, if the other experts are correct, no one wants to worry needlessly for years about whether or not exposure to dioxin has sentenced him or her to an early death or his or her child to permanent impairment.

Many thousands of Americans have been exposed to dioxin: chemical workers who manufactured a widely used herbicide; veterans of jungle warfare in Vietnam; farmers, agricultural, and forestry workers; people who lived near areas of herbicide use; the residents of Times Beach, Missouri, whose streets were sprayed with dioxin-containing oil, and consumers of fish from contaminated waters. Worldwide, other thousands of chemical industry, forestry, and agricultural workers, as well as people living near chemical plants and areas of herbicide use have been exposed. Many of those people, suffering from ill health, claim that dioxin caused their diseases as well as birth defects in their children. Many others worry that those afflictions are going to strike them as a result of exposure.

Those claims and fears have caused scientists and public health officials to carry out expensive and time-consuming studies of the health of dioxin-exposed people around the world. I discuss those studies and the controversies that have greeted their results, which generally do not support the claims made about dioxin causing disease and birth defects.

Almost from the beginning of public concern about dioxin, it was more than simply a health issue. Our government was concerned that use of dioxin-containing Agent Orange in Vietnam would be seen as chemical warfare, and it was. Both dioxin and Agent Orange are the subject of court cases here and in other countries; Federal and State regulatory agencies have eliminated from commerce the herbicide that was largely responsible for dioxin being spread in the environment and imposed strict measures to reduce exposures to residual dioxin; Congress has considered and passed legislation to compensate some veterans who may have been harmed by Agent Orange exposure. I discuss those controversies and decisions and what they mean for future claims about dioxin's health effects and how they may influence future research about the chemical. This book is intended to inform, and I think that the reader who is unsatisfied with bombardments of undigested and unanalyzed information will find it useful in formulating his or her own opinions and conclusions.

My job at the Office of Technology Assessment (OTA), the technical research arm of the United States Congress, has involved me in the Agent Orange issue since December 1979, and as OTA's representative on the White House Agent Orange Working Group, I have been abreast of research about dioxin since early 1980. I was working full-time at OTA while writing this book and my superiors approved my doing it, but it was written on my own time, and the conclusions and opinions expressed in it are my own and not necessarily those of OTA.

Many people contributed to this book. Hellen Gelband, my friend and colleague at OTA, wrote large parts of Chapters 7 and 8, and talked many hours with me as I waded through the dioxin literature and sifted my thoughts and conclusions. Scores of scientists talked with me, answering specific questions, supplying information, and expressing interest in this book.

Linda Regan, my editor, educated me about writing trade books and pushed me along. She chided me about being too academic, identified inconsistencies, and made many suggestions about style. Where the book is a pleasure to read, she can take much of the credit.

Finally, my family encouraged and humored me when I had little time for them. Lee, my wife, was unfailingly patient, upbeat, and confident. Our children, Laura and Barry, were always cooperative in using the computer for their homework and games at times I did not need it.

MICHAEL GOUGH

CONTENTS

1. Dioxin, a Prevalent Problem   13

2. Nobody Wanted Dioxin   27

3. Agent Orange and Vietnam   43

4. What We Know about Agent Orange and Veterans' Health   63

5. What We May Learn about Agent Orange and Veterans' Health   89

6. Agent Orange and Birth Defects   105

7. Dioxin in Missouri   121

8. 2,4,5-T: The United States' Disappearing Herbicide   137

9. Seveso: High-Level Environmental Exposure   149

10. The Nitro Explosion   157

11. Industrial Exposures to Dioxin   173

12. Company Behavior in the Face of Dioxin Exposures   183

13. Dioxin and Specific Cancers   193

14. Animal Tests of Dioxin Toxicity   201

15. Dioxin Decisions   221

16. The Present and the Future   237

    Appendix. Calculation of the Amount of Dioxin Exposure
              of a Person Standing under a Ranch Hand
              Spray Mission   259

    Notes   263

    Index   281

CHAPTER 1

DIOXIN, A PREVALENT PROBLEM

Toxic chemicals in the environment seem an especially unfair part of life. They go undetected for years while people walk and live on the land that these chemicals have contaminated, drink water in which they have dissolved, and breathe air containing their vapors. It seems even more unfair when children are exposed. We value children as our future; they appear more vulnerable than "tougher" adults and are very much less able to do something about environmental toxins. Their very innocence makes them seem more sensitive to toxic substances, and they have more years for the toxins to work on them.

A discovery that children may have been exposed to dioxin is certainly newsworthy. Such a discovery was made at a national campsite for Boy Scouts, and draw attention it did—at a national level. Some of the 32,000 Boy Scouts who attended the 1981 National Jamboree at the Army's Fort A. P. Hill, Virginia, slept in tents 150 feet away from a shed. On November 9, 1984, the Army announced that the shed and surrounding area were contaminated* with dioxin. Chances were small that any boy actually came into contact with dioxin, however; not only had the Scouts tented some distance from the contaminated site, but a fence between their tent site and the shed reduced opportunities for the Scouts to wander into the contaminated area.

---

*"Contaminated" means that a substance is present in an unwanted place. It does not necessarily mean that the substance is a threat to health.

Nevertheless, the November announcement raised the specter of possible cancer and other serious health effects in the exposed Scouts. The Assistant Secretary of the Army for Installations and Logistics, whose job entails, among other things, calculating how many missile sites are needed and where to locate them, met with officials of the Boy Scouts of America to tell them that the exposure during the Jamboree was "not great enough to pose a health hazard."[1]

Dr. Barry H. Rumack, Director of the Rocky Mountain Poison Center in Denver, disagreed with the Army's evaluation. "Dioxin is probably one of the most toxic chemicals known in the world," he warned. He urged those who attended the Jamboree to see a physician as soon as possible and to continue to be examined and monitored by doctors for several years.[2] He further criticized Army and Boy Scout officials, who "would like this issue to go away. Their way to make it go away is to say there's no problem."[3] Dr. Rumack also pointed out that concentrations of dioxin 150 feet from the shed were three times higher than the maximum level that is generally accepted as safe. According to measurements made by the Army and the Environmental Protection Agency (EPA), the dioxin that escaped from the shed was found downhill from it, and the Scouts camped uphill or on the level with the shed, where there was no contamination.

Dr. Rumack's suggestions had immediate effects. Worried parents flooded Boy Scout national headquarters with inquiries and, probably, physicians with requests for examinations. Dr. Rumack's statement certainly increased levels of fear and concern. Beyond that, it is difficult to see that he accomplished anything. In fact, it is possible that no Scout was exposed and it is almost beyond the realm of the possible that any Scout was exposed to sufficient dioxin to cause an effect detectable to a physician. Assuming the extreme unlikelihood that some Scout was exposed to enough dioxin to cause cancer, that dreaded disease would not be apparent until years after exposure. What were physicians to look for in the Scouts?

Parents who hauled their children off to a doctor for examination might be reassured for the short term by being told that the child was healthy. But what can the physician say about the chance of cancer 20 years in the future? Perhaps silently cursing the man who suggested the cancer threat, the physician would have to explain the limits of examinations to predict the future. If the examining physician was up to date on the burgeoning literature about dioxin, the Scout's parents could be told that the evidence for dioxin causing cancer in humans is not regarded as convincing by most experts who have studied exposed people. Besides, if it has actually caused cancer, it did so in people exposed to thousands or millions of times as much dioxin as the Scouts experienced.

Such a physician would have to be both well informed and patient. Downplaying dioxin's toxicity would probably open the door to a long discussion, with the parents making repeated references to experts who have warned of terrible consequences of exposure no matter how small. The parents still might be reassured. If so, fine. If not, they might look for another physician, one whose opinions parallel the people who warn about possible cancer.

The Army, responsible for conditions at Fort A. P. Hill, tried to respond to inquiries and concerns of Scouts and National Guard and Army Reserve troops who had bivouacked for short periods of time near the shed as well as those of other visitors to the fort. It released a statement called "Information for Parents of Scouts and Fort A. P. Hill Visitors" on November 16, 1984:

> . . . our findings thus far indicate that these very low levels of dioxin contamination are confined to a small area. This, coupled with the short exposure time (two weeks or less), show there is no likelihood of a health hazard. An independent assessment by the Centers for Disease Control supports this conclusion.[4]

While I agree with the Army's analysis, many people greeted it with skepticism or disbelief. Members of Congress, environmental organizations, and the public often criticize agencies of the Federal government for slowness in cleaning up toxic substances in the environment. Statements denying that suspect chemicals pose a health risk are common responses to such charges. The Army's statement fits that mold. I think such statements are distrusted, disregarded, or at least downgraded for two reasons. For one, resolutions of toxic incidents are seldom reported. If the government or a private agency subsequently shows that there was, in fact, little or no risk, that finding is not newsworthy, and the public may remember only that the risk was discovered and that the government did nothing. A more general reason is distrust of the government.

There is a certain irony in the Army's citing the Centers for Disease Control (CDC) as support for the conclusion that exposures at Fort A. P. Hill were not a threat to health. When Dr. Rumack said that dioxin concentrations at the fort exceeded generally accepted levels, he compared the levels there to the level that the CDC had declared unsafe at Times Beach, Missouri. The CDC is quick to point out that "safe" levels differ depending on circumstances.[5] For instance, at Times Beach, the CDC selected a level that would result in no more than a one in a million chance of developing cancer if a person lived there for 70 years. Since the Boy Scouts were at the Jamboree only two weeks, their exposure could be higher without creating a comparable risk. More to the point, unless the Scouts crossed the fence, they would not have come in contact with dioxin at all. Such statements that the "acceptable" level from Times Beach may not be applicable in all situations can easily and understandably be ignored. Americans are an impatient people, eager to get on with it, to solve the problem. We would like to have an acceptable level—a magic number—as a touchstone for deciding when an action should be taken.

Anyone who wanted to believe the Army's and CDC's reassurances would have had his credulity strained by the actions of the Environmental Protection Agency (EPA). The picture below, from *The New York Times*[6] two weeks after the Army's announcement, shows EPA workers togged out in "moon suits" to prevent any contact with any amount of dioxin, no matter how minute. How can the picture do anything but throw doubt on the Army's and the CDC's analysis that "there is no likelihood of a health hazard"? The picture cannot be reconciled even with

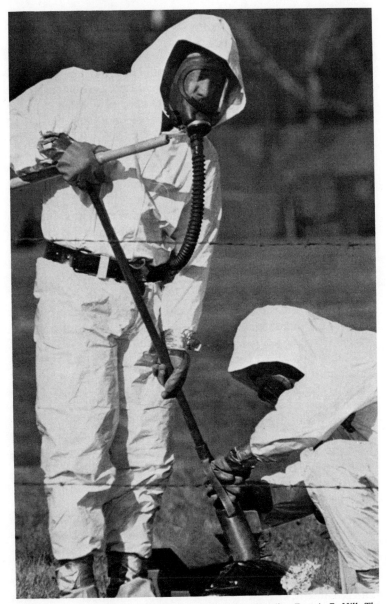

Workers from the Environmental Protection Agency sample soil at Fort A. P. Hill. The picture appeared 13 days after the Army announced that there was "no likelihood of a health hazard" for Boy Scouts who had camped nearby. Source: Wide World.

a sentence in the *Times*'s picture caption saying that "medical officials have said they [the Scouts] could not have been exposed to the dioxin long enough to be harmed." "Cavalier" is a mild word to describe a government that dresses its workers in moon suits to collect their samples in minutes or hours and that, at an earlier time, says through the Army and CDC, "Don't worry, the boys were there for only a couple of weeks."

The Fort A. P. Hill dioxin story has a happy ending. The Army's letter to the parents of all the Scouts explained that there was little risk, and the Boy Scouts of America hired an independent engineering firm to verify that the government's measurements were accurate. After determining the limits of the contamination, the Army and EPA scraped up the contaminated soil and hauled it away to a disposal site. Then the excavated area was covered with fresh soil, and the 1985 Jamboree opened on schedule in late July.

Despite the successful resolution, the government's early actions appeared, at best, confused, incompetent, and uncertain; at worst, deceitful, schizophrenic, and even uncaring about its citizens' health. The Fort A. P. Hill dioxin episode is an example of the too frequently conflicting words and actions of the government and other authorities about environmental toxins. It is an extreme example because the exposed people were children. The importance of that is illustrated by the Army's information paper saying, "While some of the Jamboree staff used the building for storing equipment, it was not used by or readily accessible to the scout youth at the Jamboree." Hence, the Army treated the leaders as less vulnerable and their exposures as less important.

The example is also extreme because dioxin is not an "average" environmental toxin. It is number one. Of course, generalized fear of "chemicals" causing grave health effects contributes to dioxin's notoriety, but that cannot explain dioxin's prominence. Citizens and public health officials tolerate other cancer-causing chemicals in the air, water, food, and soil with much less overt concern. Who even knows the name of the "second most toxic chemical," much less worries about it?

Dioxin, for a number of valid reasons, is news. It was present in millions of pounds of Agent Orange that were sprayed in Vietnam, and veterans of that war complain that it is causing diseases and birth defects. That war in itself tore at our country's sense of self and mission, leaving unhealed wounds. Is its final irony to be that its veterans are condemned to early death and their children to a legacy of chemically caused defects and diseases? Whatever a person thought about our country's participation in that war, surely no one wants a plague of illness and physically and mentally impaired children. And if Agent Orange left those consequences, we, as a nation, owe compensation to the veterans and their families. Despite veterans' claims, however, evidence for Agent Orange exposure having caused any or all of a panoply of diseases and birth defects remains unconvincing. At the same time, the claims and arguments keep dioxin in the public eye, contributing to its importance as a public health issue.

Unknown numbers of people came into contact with dioxin when dioxin-containing herbicides were used throughout this country. EPA proceedings in the late 1970s highlighted claims that herbicide spraying of forests in the Pacific Northwest caused miscarriages among women living there. In 1983, United States manufacture of the herbicides ended.

Swedish scientists examined the occurrence of a rare form of cancer and discovered that lumberjacks were five or six times as likely to have the disease as men in other occupations. According to the scientists' investigation, the lumberjacks were frequently exposed to dioxin-containing herbicides. Subsequent studies showed that workers exposed to the herbicides in another region of Sweden were also afflicted by the rare cancer far more often than expected. Furthermore, a more common cancer that strikes many more people was found at greater than expected frequencies in dioxin-exposed workers.

These observations of human health effects are reinforced by studies in laboratory animals that convincingly show dioxin to cause cancer, birth defects, and abortions. Results of those studies are frequently cited in the press, repeating the chemical's name and properties before the public.

However, the dread effects attributed to dioxin occur frequently in humans: About 20% of the United States population dies from cancer, a large fraction, perhaps a majority, of all pregnancies end in spontaneous abortions (often so early that the woman is unaware that she had been pregnant), and 3% of all live-born babies suffer from a serious structural birth defect. Such disasters are almost always without explanation. With no information about what caused the tragedy, it is reasonable to look at known toxic agents as possibly being responsible. The well-publicized toxicity of dioxin, in combination with information that there had been any opportunity for exposure, can lead to conclusions and contentions that it caused any of a large number of health problems.

As is illustrated by events surrounding the Scout Jamboree at Fort A. P. Hill, demonstrated disease is not required for dioxin to have an effect on perceptions about health and disease. In the absence of any apparent adverse effects, knowledge of dioxin's toxicity, coupled with the thought that people might have had contact with it, sets off a wave of fear that healthy people, unknowingly exposed, are at elevated risk of future disease.

The dioxin contamination at Fort A. P. Hill did not come from some large-scale chemical program. Instead, it was spills or leaks from two drums of herbicides in the storage shed. Any garage, basement, farm building, or shed used by homeowners, golf course operators, herbicide applicators, farmers, or anyone else to store dioxin-containing herbicides might be similarily contaminated. Unlike the EPA's sample takers, who were fully protected against contact with the chemical and who were in the contaminated area for a few minutes or hours, homeowners, farmers, and others may work unprotected for hours at a time, day after day, in a contaminated environment. Should the EPA dispatch its moon-suited workers around the country to look for dioxin contamination wherever herbicides were stored or used? Economically, that is impossible. The EPA does not have the resources. That practical response still leaves unanswered the larger question of whether or not people are at greatly increased risk of cancer and other maladies because of exposures to levels of dioxin comparable to that at Fort A. P. Hill. The answer is no.

That opinion should draw an immediate response from

people who are more worried about the health effects of dioxin: "We have to act now to reduce exposures. We know from limited human experience and convincing animal studies that dioxin is terribly toxic, and if we wait, the proof of its human toxicity will be increased cancer and birth defects."

I cannot overstate the difficulties inherent in designing and executing studies to produce hard and fast answers to questions about how dioxin or any other environmental pollutant affects humans. Furthermore, the results we possess are subject to differing interpretations. Some results lead to conclusions that there are associations between exposure to dioxin and particular diseases. Other apparently contradictory studies do not find associations. In some cases, the "negative" study was too "weak" to detect the "positive" association seen in the "stronger" study. Any of a number of factors can contribute to a weak study. If the usual rate of occurrence of a disease is 1 case in 100 people, and a study examines 25 people, the rate would have to be 4 times normal to be detected. Timing can be a problem. Cancer is a disease of middle and old age and is thought to occur decades after exposure to a carcinogen. To examine a group of people 1 or 5 or 10 years after their exposure and find no excess cancer cases is not convincing evidence. Part of the confusion about possible health effects of dioxin stems from mixing together the results of weak studies that in reality do not support any conclusions with results from other, stronger studies. Other studies are flatly contradictory. For instance, the excess of a rare cancer that was reported in Swedish lumberjacks exposed to dioxin was not found in forestry workers in Finland or in herbicide sprayers in New Zealand. In those cases, detailed examination of the studies is necessary to decide why they differ and which is more likely to be correct.

To study the possible human health effects of chemicals appears, at first glance, deceptively simple. It would seem an easy task to study populations of exposed people by examining their health and medical records or by interviewing them to see if they are suffering unusual numbers or types of diseases as compared to unexposed people. Unfortunately, complications plague such analyses. Disparities in access to medical care, diagnoses, and reporting of disease among doctors and geographical areas complicate the process. Determining that a person was exposed to a particular chemical is a difficult undertaking unless the person was exposed on the job; yet workplaces are fraught with multitudes of chemicals, making it difficult to ascertain which exposure caused the ill health. Furthermore, it is almost always impossible to quantify exposures, to know which people were exposed to large amounts of the substance and which were exposed to much less. Hence epidemiology—the study of the distribution of human illnesses and their causes—can be an uncertain and costly undertaking.

Furthermore, scientific knowledge of the health effects of dioxin (and other chemicals) on humans is so limited that we must rely on tests on animals to make predictions about human effects. Then scientists are saddled with the problem that measurements of dioxin's toxicity vary immensely depending on which animal is used to test it. For instance, the amount of dioxin necessary to kill one hamster would kill 5000 guinea pigs. Similarly, although there is convincing evidence that dioxin causes cancer, abortions, and birth defects in animals, the application of that information to humans is subject to dispute, especially when it has been demonstrated that some results obtained in studies on rats differ from some obtained on mice. If the tests do not agree between those relatively closely related animals, how can they be used to predict human effects?

Some proportion of the hundreds of millions of dollars allocated to scientific investigations of dioxin is being spent on animal studies. Some will sharpen our knowledge of how dioxin works at the molecular level, and may provide powerful information for making decisions about associations between the chemical and disease. At the same time, animal studies leave many people cold. We already know that dioxin causes illnesses in animals and then kills them. What more do we need to know from animals?

Perhaps the only thing certain about the results of animal tests is that the terms "uncertain" and "uncertainty" will crop up whenever they are used to make predictions about humans. In the business of predicting human risk, where a person sits or works is often predictive of what position he will take in a controversy—although this is hotly denied by participants on all sides. Manufacturers may be convinced of the safety of their products because of data or because they choose to ignore reports of their products causing adverse effects. On the other side, public interest groups may be convinced that a product is hazardous because of other facts or because of different interpretations of the same facts. Or the latter may lump all chemicals together, expecting such unattainably high standards for safety that essentially all chemicals would be considered a hazard of some kind or another.

Additional scientific inquiry may resolve some of the differing interpretations and sway some opinions, but science is slow. Moreover, the process of science itself is unsure; sometimes studies simply "don't work" and fail to provide the solid answers so desperately sought.

Science and society, in wanting to resolve difficult questions about toxic substances and other hazards, have fostered a new discipline called "risk assessment." Sold by its proponents as a rigorous undertaking that does not depend on opinions or, at least, spells out opinions, risk assessment is offered as a unique tool for making decisions on controversies such as dioxin. Its luminous promise is that it will produce an objective, quantitative estimate of dioxin's risk. That estimate can then be compared with other estimates to place dioxin in a proper perspective within a catalogue of risks that we now contemplate, regulate, or tolerate.

Risk assessment is not all that it is sometimes cracked up to be, however. It is not like addition, where the rules guarantee that everyone who knows how to carry out the manipulations will get the same answer to a given problem. Instead, different risk assessors confronted with the same problem may well produce different results. When there are many facts and opinions, some may be ignored in analyses. Some are ignored for good reason, but one person's "good reason" may be dismissed as "valueless" or "value-laden" opinion by someone else. The selection of what data to consider and what to ignore profoundly influences the course of risk assessment, as does the selection of a "mathematical model" to estimate risks when few data are available. As is well known in the risk-assessment trade, risk estimates for a single substance may vary by factors of tens, hundreds, thousands, or more depending on the data chosen and models used.

Most scientists take a tolerant view of risk assessment, warts and all. To be believed, risk assessors must lay out the data they considered, how they analyzed the data, and how they arrived at their judgments. This process of "showing your work" greatly facilitates understanding, and it is worlds better than an individual's proclamations that calculations have been done and that they show dioxin is a terrible risk or no risk at all. In such a case there is nothing to examine.

When the epidemiological studies have been completed and the animal tests finished and the risk assessors have done their job, we should have an estimate (or estimates) of the risk posed by dioxin. So what? Is the risk small enough to put up with or so great that we should spend time and money to reduce it? These are not scientific questions. In a democracy, they are questions to be answered by citizens, and in our country, we count on the courts and political system to provide answers.

Because it is more than a scientific question and problem, dioxin invites political and legal controversies, involving sick and worried people who are petitioning the government for compensation or help in reducing risk and who are suing other people for damages. In our society, we can resolve such controversies by electing people to office, influencing particular lawmakers, relying on regulatory agencies to make a decision, or going to court. In the case of dioxin, all these avenues have been employed by parties on various sides of the issue. However, all the legal and political approaches have drawn on science. Claims of damage or threats to health have been buttressed by references to epidemiological and animal studies. Estimates of possible harm have been drawn directly from risk assessment. The dioxin issue in the courts, legislatures, and regulatory agencies, so far at least, has not been divorced from scientific investigation and results.

The intertwining of legal, political, and scientific processes in efforts to resolve the controversies about dioxin has thrown policymakers and scientists together. It is an uneasy alliance, strained by suspicion on each side of the other's methods for gathering facts, synthesizing information, understanding problems, and developing solutions.

A scientific fact differs from a legal fact; the former is not accepted as "proved" unless it is verifiable by another scientist in another location and if repeated tests fail to prove it false; the latter is "proved" if a preponderance of opinion says that it took place. Many scientists can only regard with horror the idea that judges and juries can decide questions about the cause of a disease when their own approach to coming to conclusions requires years of diligent inquiry. The patience of decision-makers is strained by scientists' insistence on more time, but it is burst asunder when, at the end of their studies, scientists still remain uncertain about questions of causality.

Some legal decisions have already been made about dioxin. A Canadian court denied the petition of a group of landowners who objected to spraying of nearby forests with herbicides containing traces of dioxin. It stated that the low levels would cause no harm. Veterans who claimed harm from Agent Orange reached a settlement with manufacturers of that herbicide, and the judge in the case expressed his opinion that the veterans' claims were not valid. A jury decided that the lives of workers had not been threatened even though they had been exposed to high levels of dioxin during an explosion and its aftermath.

Currently, few awards are being made to plaintiffs claiming harm from dioxin. Let us assume that that trend continues but that subsequent studies show there is a relationship between exposure and disease. What will the victors and losers in the court battle do? Alternatively, what if awards are made to plaintiffs who claim they were harmed and subsequently completed studies provide no scientific underpinnings for causal relationships between exposure to dioxin and disease? Will the courts reopen? The questions could become more and more complex.

State and Federal legislators have responded to veterans' claims that their illnesses are associated with exposure to Agent

Orange. First, they ordered studies to investigate the claims. Now they have moved to providing some direct benefits for Vietnam veterans. Congress has directed the Veterans Administration (VA) hospitals to grant Vietnam veterans priority if there is a shortage of VA beds or treatment facilities. In the fall of 1984, Congress passed and President Reagan signed a law directing the VA to compensate any Vietnam veteran who suffers from either of two specific and rare diseases that developed within one year of leaving Vietnam. The presumption behind the law is that the two diseases are associated with exposure to Agent Orange during the war.

The Office of Science and Technology Policy in the White House estimates that the Federal government spent one billion dollars on dioxin research in 1985. Without doubt, these expenditures and ones still to be made will increase our store of information about dioxin. However, they will almost certainly find no significant human health problems resulting from exposures to dioxin in the environment or from exposures of veterans to Agent Orange; the reasons for this we shall see later. One of the problems we face is saying yes or no to new studies. If problems are not shown to exist, what do we do? Conclude that the studies were not the best that can be done and start new ones? Or conclude that we have looked hard enough and that we will not find anything more?

Before any judgments can be made, we must first look at what dioxin is and how it came to be the problem it is.

CHAPTER 2

NOBODY WANTED DIOXIN

From the time of their introduction, asbestos and the pesticides EDB, lindane, and chlordane were enthusiastically received; soon they were used in huge quantities. The public considered asbestos desirable for its flame-retardant properties and EDB, lindane, and chlordane desirable for controlling pests that were destroying food and property. Entering commerce as "good actors"—useful for particular jobs—they became "bad actors"— pollutants or toxic chemicals—once scientists and physicians discovered that they were a threat to human health.

Both benefits and liabilities are bound to crop up during debates about asbestos, EDB, lindane, and chlordane. Surely many people are grateful that asbestos saved them from a fiery death, especially sailors who were on ships that would have burned faster and more intensely when shells, bombs, or torpedos hit them. And when it comes to firefighters, there is no substitute for asbestos when fighting the hottest fires. In the case of citrus fruit and grain growers and shippers, EDB, by reducing loss to insects, permitted lower prices and improved the quality and appearance of their products. Similarly, many homeowners appreciated the usefulness of chlordane and lindane in protecting their houses from termites. For those products, all of which were later shown to present risks to human health, real benefits were derived from their use.

Dioxin* is different, however. It has always been a pollutant

---

*For the purposes of this book, "dioxin" will be used to refer to the chemical 2,3,7,8-tetrachlorobenzene-*p*-dioxin, which is the most toxic of the 75 chlori-

or contaminant in the strictest sense. No one ever manufactured and sold dioxin for use in general commerce or the environment. Except for a handful of chemists who make minute amounts for research purposes, no one has ever made it intentionally. It was not sprayed into the environment to check pests or to improve crop productivity. No one has ever argued that it has any benefits whatsoever.

Dioxin came into existence as an unavoidable by-product in the manufacture of other useful products. It also derives from fires of various sources. Most attention centers on the dioxin that is a by-product in the synthesis of the chemical trichlorophenol,[†] through which process hundreds of pounds of dioxin have been made. The Dow Chemical Company, in a series of papers, has pushed the idea that another major source of dioxin is fires. According to that theory, burning a variety of substances—e.g., wood, garbage, plastics—produces dioxin that filters into the environment; hence, the implication is that at least some of the dioxin in our environment can be laid to fires and not to chemical manufacturers.

In reality, it is impossible to tell the difference between molecules of dioxin made by chemical manufacturers and ones produced by fires. Given equal exposures, dioxin from either source poses an equal risk to human health. Although there are controversies about the relative importance of both sources of dioxin, almost everything we know about the health effects of dioxin was learned by studying people exposed to the manufactured chemical, not because it is more dangerous, but because industrial exposures were higher. It is also easier to identify

---

nated dioxins. This usage, while imprecise, is consistent with the use of "dioxin" in the news media, where it almost always refers to 2,3,7,8,-tetrachlorobenzene-*p*-dioxin. Dioxin is an unavoidable by-product in the making of the herbicide 2,4,5-T and as an unwanted contaminant of that herbicide present in Agent Orange.

[†]"Trichlorophenol" will be used to refer to the chemical 2,4,5-trichlorophenol, which is important in its role as a precursor to 2,4,5-T and some other pesticides. It is impossible to synthesize trichlorophenol without making dioxin as a by-product, so trichlorophenol and all chemicals subsequently made from it contain traces of dioxin.

workers in trichlorophenol and 2,4,5-T pesticide factories for study than to locate members of the general population who have been exposed. In fact, a bit of clever medical detective work following an outbreak of industrial dermatitis, not routine chemical research and analysis, was what discovered dioxin in trichlorophenol.

In 1957 in Germany, Dr. Karl Schulz of the University of Hamburg examined a chemical plant worker's skin disease. He recognized the disease as chloracne—a persistent skin disease—and subsequently found several other workers from the same plant who had developed the disease. As a dermatologist who examined chemical workers, Dr. Schulz was familiar with chloracne and able to recognize it. The disease is so uncommon outside the chemical industry that most physicians never see a case.

In its mildest form, chloracne resembles teen-age acne. But on closer inspection, it differs in that the blackheads and cysts cluster in two locations: appearing in a crescent pattern outside of and under the eyes and behind the ears, the so-called "eyeglass" or "spectacle" distribution. In more pronounced cases, pustules, pus-containing spots, erupt and spread across the rest of the face, neck and shoulders, genitalia, chest, back, and lower trunk in that order. There are limits to the spread of the disease, and the eruptions only rarely reach the hands, feet, and legs. In some cases, the disease causes an excess of skin pigmentation, giving the skin, especially the face, a gray cast.

Severe chloracne is a far worse disease than common acne. The face can be so covered with blackheads and pimples that afflicted people are too self-conscious to show themselves in public. Worse, the spots from chloracne can cause scarring and result in some permanent disfigurement.

Seen almost exclusively in chemical industry workers, chloracne was first described in Germany in 1895. The name, a telescoping of "chlorine acne," was given to the disease because chlorine gas, widely used in chemistry, was initially and incorrectly thought to be its cause.

Further research revealed that a class of chemicals called chlorinated aromatic hydrocarbons cause the disease. Hydrocarbons are a vast array of chemicals that contain hydrogen and carbon. As their name suggests, many aromatic hydrocarbons have distinct smells (because of the nature of chemical bonds within the molecule). Everyone knows the smell of at least one aromatic hydrocarbon, naphthalene, from which mothballs are made. In chlorinated aromatic hydrocarbons, some or all of the hydrogen atoms of the chemical are replaced by chlorine atoms. We have already mentioned two chlorinated aromatic hydrocarbons by name: dioxin and trichlorophenol. Others that are essential to this discussion are the herbicides 2,4-D (2,4-dichlorophenoxyacetic acid) and 2,4,5-T* (2,4,5-trichlorophenoxyacetic acid).

Dr. Schulz suspected that the aromatic hydrocarbon trichlorophenol, manufactured in the Boehringer plant that employed the chemical workers, caused the chloracne. He availed himself of a standard animal test to investigate his suspicion. In his laboratory, he applied highly purified and, separately, less purified ("commercial-grade") trichlorophenol to the inside surfaces of rabbits' ears. Although the purified chemical caused no reaction, the commercial-grade caused eruptions similar to chloracne on the rabbit ears. The conclusion was obvious: Some impurity present in the relatively impure commercial-grade chemical caused the chloracne.

It is not surprising that commercial-grade trichlorophenol was contaminated with other chemicals. Chemical companies routinely make different grades of chemicals for different uses. For instance, commercial-grade trichlorophenol can be processed into the pesticide 2,4,5-T or sold to another firm that makes 2,4,5-T. However, commercial-grade chemicals are notorious for being "dirty," that is, containing other chemicals as "impurities," the identities of which may or may not be known. As long as the impurities in commercial-grade trichlorophenol do not interfere with the reaction necessary to make 2,4,5-T, the trichlorophenol manufacturer will probably not bother to purify them away. Purification costs money, and if it does not improve

---

*From this point on, "2,4,5-T" will be used to refer to the herbicide of that name and to the herbicide "Silvex." They are chemically very closely related, their mode of action as herbicides is the same, both are made from trichlorophenol, and both contain dioxin.

the market for the chemical, what is the incentive to do it? Knowing that a health threat is associated with an impurity can be a powerful incentive, but in the mid-1950s, little was known about the impurities in trichlorophenol, and nothing about dioxin. Of course, much more is known now, and although trichlorophenol is no longer made in the United States, trichlorophenol currently manufactured elsewhere is much "cleaner" than the commercial-grade chemical tested by Dr. Schulz.

Dr. Schulz had access to highly purified trichlorophenol because manufacturers often prepare small amounts of more highly purified products. The chemicals "cleaned up" to higher and higher purity are used and sold for research purposes and for studying the properties of the "pure" chemical.

George Sorge, a chemist employed by Boehringer, supplied Dr. Schulz with a number of chemicals thought to contaminate commercial-grade trichlorophenol. Each was tested on rabbits' ears, and none caused the chloracne-like disease. The experiments left the chemist and dermatologist with perplexing results; they knew that something in commercial-grade trichlorophenol caused chloracne, but they could not pinpoint what it was.

There the matter lay until a laboratory accident occurred while chemists in Dr. W. Sandermann's laboratory were synthesizing a new substance for trial as a wood preservative. The new product had been dried to a powder in laboratory apparatus, and when a laboratory assistant opened the container, some of the dry material blew into his face. He soon developed chloracne as shown in the photograph below. Fortunately for our understanding of dioxin, the assistant sought treatment at Dr. Schulz's dermatology clinic.

The dermatologist informed his colleague, the chemist Sorge, about the accident, which they saw as a key to unlock the puzzle of what chemical caused chloracne in the trichlorophenol workers. Suspecting that the cause of the laboratory assistant's eruptions might very well be identical to the one in commercial-grade trichlorophenol, they reanalyzed the trichlorophenol. The chemical that had been synthesized in Dr. Sandermann's labora-

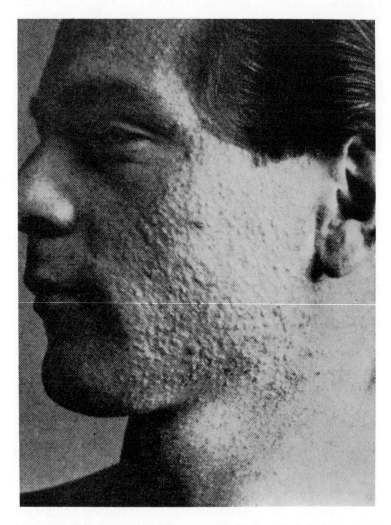

Chloracne on a laboratory worker's face. Source: Alvin Young, who obtained it from Prof. K. H. Schulz, Dermatologische Klinik, Universität Hamburg.

tory and that Sorge found in trichlorophenol were identical. Both were dioxin.[1]

To be certain of this finding, Dr. Schulz tested dioxin not only on rabbits' ears but also on his own forearm; chloracne appeared in both places. In 1985, 28 years after the experiment, scars from chloracne still remain on his left forearm.

The fruitful collaboration between Schulz and Sorge provided the first information about the health effects of dioxin. Moreover, it brought about a happy ending for Sorge's employer, Boehringer. Without knowing the details of the chemistry that produced dioxin, Sorge intuited that lowering the temperatures used in making trichlorophenol would reduce dioxin formation. In keeping with this hunch, he saw to it that production temperatures were lowered. Though his modifications did not completely eliminate dioxin from trichlorophenol, they reduced its concentration sufficiently to prevent chloracne, thus ridding the Boehringer workforce of the disease.

Chloracne has particular importance as a disease because scientists accept without reservation that it is caused by dioxin. However, since other chlorinated aromatic hydrocarbons can cause the disease, chloracne is not a certain indicator of dioxin exposure. The matter thus becomes even more confusing. Not all people who work in areas contaminated with dioxin develop chloracne, in part because of differing sensitivity to dioxin and in part because of different levels of exposure. Hence, if a person has been in a situation where exposure to dioxin is possible, and chloracne does develop, dioxin exposure is a near certainty. The "chloracne, yes—exposure, yes" agreement does not, however, have a reciprocal of "chloracne, no—exposure, no" because we know that some workers who have been exposed to dioxin do not come down with the disease.

Most people already know that Agent Orange was contaminated with dioxin, but what other herbicides are contaminated? Let us suppose that we gave to a thousand urban dwellers cards with the following names listed on them:

Agent Orange
Silvex
2,4-D
2,4,5-T

We would then ask each person to check off which ones were the names of herbicides. Agent Orange would be ticked off most frequently because news accounts often identify it as an herbicide. Many people would also know that Agent Orange was contaminated with dioxin. If we were to give the same card to a thousand rural dwellers and ask them the same questions, many would tick off all four names as herbicides. They would have learned about Agent Orange from news stories and veterans' accounts, and they would know about the other three because Silvex, 2,4-D, and 2,4,5-T are (or more correctly "were" in the case of Silvex and 2,4,5-T) commonly used herbicides in farming and forestry. They would probably know that Silvex and 2,4,5-T are contaminated with dioxin.

To understand how people are exposed to dioxin, we need to know where it comes from, how it enters the environment, and where it goes. Consider Agent Orange, a 50:50 mixture of 2,4-D and 2,4,5-T, which was purchased by the Defense Department to defoliate enemy territory and destroy enemy crops in Vietnam. All the 2,4,5-T contained dioxin because all of it was made from trichlorophenol, which cannot be produced without some dioxin being carried along as a by-product. However little or much dioxin is in the trichlorophenol, and levels were much higher in the 1960s during the heyday of 2,4,5-T production for Agent Orange use, it is carried along through processing into other chemicals. Workers along the process can be exposed, as well as herbicide users and people where it is used.

People who work in manufacturing trichlorophenol can be exposed to dioxin through "explosions" or "runaway reactions" or "events." Each of these terms means the same thing, a small-scale explosion, but workers and their representatives, claiming damages to health, choose the first word, whereas owners of chemical plants and their representatives, denying or downplaying adverse effects, will use one of the less loaded words. In any case, trichlorophenol explosions are more akin to a pressure cooker blowing its lid than to a bomb going off. When the explosion occurs, the chemicals in the reaction vessel are forced into the workrooms, exposing everyone to fumes, liquids, and solid particles containing dioxin. More mundane industrial exposures are called "leaks." If connections of the equipment in the chemical plant are not tight, enough trichlorophenol and dioxin may seep into the plant, generally as fumes, to cause chloracne. Moreover, every routine service and repair of equipment exposes workers to any liquid or solid residues remaining in the equipment.

Employees making 2,4,5-T can be exposed to dioxin as it is carried along in trichlorophenol to be converted to the herbicide. The actual synthesis of 2,4,5-T has no effect on dioxin; thus, dioxin that enters the reaction ends up in the herbicide.

"Formulators" are workers whose job it is to mix pesticides together or to mix pesticides with other chemicals to make the pesticide easier to apply or "stickier" so that it will work better. Agent Orange formulators mixed 2,4,5-T containing dioxin with the other, closely related herbicide 2,4-D. (2,4-D is contaminated with some other forms of dioxin, but *not* with the highly toxic variety that is present in trichlorophenol and 2,4,5-T. The dioxins in 2,4-D are so much less toxic that their effects can be ignored in considering the overall toxicity of Agent Orange.)

The last occupational group to risk exposure to dioxin are "applicators" who spray to otherwise disseminate Agent Orange, 2,4,5-T, or other dioxin-contaminated pesticides into the environment. In this country, applicators sprayed 2,4,5-T in forests, croplands, and pastures to control broadleaf plants. For instance, scrubby deciduous plants can outgrow young, economically desirable evergreens and block their access to sunlight, broadleaf weeds can reduce rice crop yields, and prickly pear can prevent animals from grazing. The most famous applicators in history, however, are the pilots, air crews, and ground crews of the Air Force's "Operation Ranch Hand" who sprayed millions of pounds of Agent Orange in Vietnam.

Anyone who is in or near an area sprayed with 2,4,5-T or Agent Orange risks exposure to dioxin. Such people are not "occupationally" exposed; instead, they are "environmentally" exposed. Few, if any, environmentally exposed persons received large doses of dioxin comparable to those experienced by production workers, formulators, or applicators. Yet there is no question that the number of people who have been environmentally exposed is huge. For instance, an undoubtedly large, but unknown, fraction of the 2.8 million Vietnam veterans were exposed to Agent Orange, and considering the amounts of 2,4,5-T used in this country, other thousands or millions have had to be exposed here.

Yet there are environmental exposures more risky than incidental exposure to sprayings. When trichlorophenol is produced, "still bottoms," thick, viscous dioxin-containing materials, accumulate in the reaction vessels. The still bottoms are somewhat analogous to the sludge in the bottom of a car crankcase. Periodic cleaning out of still bottoms exposes workers to high concentrations of dioxin. In addition, still bottoms themselves present a disposal problem.

High-temperature incineration of still bottoms or any other waste can completely destroy dioxin, eliminating any risk, but other disposal techniques leave substantial exposure risks. Before society became aware that chemical wastes posed potential threats to human health, it was an accepted practice to discard chemical residues, including still bottoms, in waste dumps. Neither the safe disposal method, incineration, nor the unsafe one, dumping, generates any revenue for the company that has still bottoms to dispose of; on the contrary, both cost money.

An alternative to a manufacturer directly disposing of its wastes was to pay other businesses to haul them off and dispose of them. Sinclair Lewis said of the Chicago stockyards that they sell everything of the pig but the squeal, and business has to look for saleable items and services. With entrepreneurial spirit, some haulers found a market for still bottoms, which are dense and oily. When mixed with other oily materials, still bottoms were sold and sprayed on dirt roads and other unpaved, ungrassed areas to suppress dust. This inventive marketing idea for still bottoms introduced untold amounts of dioxin into the environment.

The Environmental Protection Agency (EPA) estimates that *80–90% of all the dioxin ever made in chemical plants ended up in still bottoms.* The EPA refuses to estimate the *amount* of dioxin that was made by manufacturers and provides no information about how much dioxin was in still bottoms or how much of the still bottoms was disposed of by incineration or dumping or used in dust suppression. We do know, however, that still bottoms have wrought havoc. To eliminate exposure to dioxin, the Federal government bought Times Beach, Missouri, because the chemical had been sprayed on roads throughout the town as part of a dust-suppression program. The Canadian government[2] estimates that over 100 pounds of dioxin lie buried in the Love Canal and more than two tons (an unbelievably large amount) in the Hyde Park Dump near Niagara Falls, New York. No one can deny that these are huge amounts; they can be compared to the total of 368 pounds[3] of dioxin sprayed in Vietnam over a six-year period. Unfortunately, we cannot estimate the magnitude of the remaining dioxin waste problem, because there is no record of the amounts of dioxin sprayed for dust suppression or buried in every dump.

The people most highly exposed to dioxin are workers in chemical manufacturing plants, and the second most highly exposed are probably formulators. Following them in exposure are workers who sprayed dioxin-containing herbicides. People who lived in or near sprayed areas are less exposed, although the number of such people is probably many times greater than the number of exposed workers. While that order of exposure would cover most situations, some Vietnam veterans claim that they were drenched with Agent Orange from airplanes. Clearly, anyone who was soaked in the stuff was significantly exposed.

Three problems plague efforts to understand dioxin's risk for humans: uncertainty about what dioxin does to human health, uncertainty about who was exposed to dioxin, and uncertainty about how much of it anyone was exposed to. Were a person to be standing under an airplane or beside a truck spraying 2,4,5-T or Agent Orange, he or she would certainly be exposed. But let us consider possible reactions to knowing that a friend had walked into an area a day after it was sprayed. Sunlight degrades dioxin, so if the sun had been shining, much or all of the dioxin would have been destroyed. That may be a comforting idea, intellectually, but if the friend later developed a disease believed to be caused by dioxin, he might be unwilling to agree that sunlight inactivates dioxin. Instead, he might claim that dioxin caused his illness and sue the applicator, formulator, or manufacturer. The people being sued, on the other hand, would argue that any exposure under those conditions was unimportant and that dioxin could not cause the disease anyway.

As widely as dioxin is distributed through manufacture and use of herbicides, consider how even more widespread it would be if it were produced by ordinary fires. Then it would be expected nearly everywhere.

In 1978, scientists at the Dow Chemical Company[4] put forth the novel idea that dioxins are formed in fires. It takes no great amount of cynicism to suggest that the idea of dioxin from fire might be a good one for Dow to pursue. That company, at that time, was manufacturing trichlorophenol, and with attention focused on dioxin's possible threat to human health, the company might have found it useful to point to other sources of the chemical. At first, Dow contended that dioxin was produced by the burning of chemical plant wastes and even by cigarettes. Scientists, however, criticized those studies on the basis that those materials were synthetic products, which might have contained dioxin before they were ever burned.

Subsequently, scientists at Dow scraped deposits from wood-burning stoves that were used in rural areas and analyzed them for dioxin.[5] Since dioxin was found in most samples, the notion that fires produced dioxin took on more credibility. However, apparently subtle differences between stoves or fuels can have a profound influence on the production of dioxin. For instance, samples from four wood stoves in New Hampshire were analyzed. Although all the wood burned in the stoves came from the same woodlot, soot samples from three stoves contained dioxin, while the other did not. The scientists who reported those findings have no explanation for the discrepancy, but rather emphasized the general finding that dioxin is produced by wood fires, and suggested that such combustion may produce more dioxin than any other source. At the same meeting where scientists from Dow reported finding dioxin in wood-burning stoves, other scientists from Environment Canada (the equivalent of the United States EPA) presented a paper[6] that said no dioxin of the type found in trichlorophenol and 2,4,5-T was present in wood-burning stoves. These direct contradictions have yet to be resolved; differences in the techniques used by different scientists may have influenced the reported results. Although Dow may not expend much more effort on fire-generated dioxin because the company no longer makes trichlorophenol and, I expect, its interest in dioxin has lessened, many other scientists are active in detailing what kinds of fires produce dioxin.

For instance, a paper prepared by the Canadian government[7] lists municipal and industrial incineration as the single greatest source of dioxin. The burning of complex mixtures of materials provides ample amounts of carbon, hydrogen, and chlorine, the right ingredients for the synthesis of dioxin. Furthermore, some incinerators burn at temperatures high enough to favor the synthesis of dioxin, yet not high enough to degrade any dioxin that is made. An obvious solution for this problem is to raise the temperature, but the temperature necessary to destroy dioxin cannot be attained in many currently used municipal incinerators. Instead of simply raising the temperature, a new incinerator may have to be built to ensure destruction of dioxin.

Taken at face value, the data about wood fires releasing dioxin into the atmosphere say that dioxin has been around as long as fire. If that is true, dioxin is not a new hazard, sprung upon us by modern industry. Moreover, forcing reductions in the amounts of chemicals that contain traces of dioxin may not be the most effective method of lowering exposures to the chemical. One might be led to believe that perhaps wood fires should be regulated.

Some simple observations should resolve questions about the significance of wood fires as a major source of dioxin. If dioxin has been produced for eons by forest fires and the like, the chemical, bound to dust particles, should have been laid down on the soil for hundreds and thousands of years. It is possible to investigate that hypothesis by drilling down into layers of undisturbed soil or sediment on lake bottoms and analyzing them for dioxin at different depths.

Isle Royale, Michigan, is located in northern Lake Superior.

Since it is a National Park, no automobiles have been allowed on it since 1940. Any industrial chemicals that reach the island must be borne in by the air. When scientists from Indiana University examined sediment from a lake on the island, they found trace amounts of dioxin in the upper layers, but steadily decreasing concentration in layers deposited before 1940.[8] Because the proportions of dioxin and other industrial chemicals in the upper layers closely parallel those seen in air samples from Washington, D.C., and St. Louis, Missouri, the scientists concluded that the chemicals originated in incinerators from far-off cities and were carried by the wind to the island.

It is widely believed that burning plastics is an important source of dioxin. United States incinerators, which are crammed with plastics from our throw-away society, typically produce higher levels of dioxin than do European incinerators. Since plastics became really important beginning in the 1940s, it is reasonable to conclude that the appearance of dioxin at Isle Royale coincides with the large-scale burning of plastic. Of course, its appearance also coincides with the beginning of large-scale production of trichlorophenol.

The steadily decreasing amounts of dioxin found in sediment that was laid down before 1940 contradict the hypothesis that wood fires have been major sources of dioxin. Wood fires have been around forever. But nothing is easy when it comes to dioxin, so it is no surprise that other scientists have found dioxin in older soils, supporting the wood-fire theory. The controversy about wood fires will continue, but other types of fires are probably more important as sources of dioxin.

Finding dioxin at Isle Royale shows two things: (1) The chemical can move long distances through the air and (2) dioxin-detection methods are sufficiently sensitive to detect truly minute amounts. The maximum concentrations of dioxin on Isle Royale were only about 4% of the level set as unsafe for lifetime exposure at Times Beach, Missouri.

Despite dioxin's being found in pristine Isle Royale, we can take comfort from reports that dioxin is not ubiquitous. The EPA has analyzed soil samples from around the United States, and dioxin is simply not detectable in some of them.[9] These observations do not disprove the fire theory, nor that dioxin can be distributed by the wind, but they at least show that it is not everywhere.

Burning coal apparently does not produce dioxin at all; analyses of smoke and ash from coal-burning power plants have failed to find dioxin. Furthermore, no dioxin was found to be emitted from a municipal incinerator that burned a mixture of refuse and coal. Coal-fueled fires can reach the very high temperatures that destroy dioxin. As a reminder that there is no such thing as a free lunch, although coal fires do not emit dioxin, there is evidence that other emissions from coal contribute to thousands of cancer deaths yearly.[10]

Scientists have not resolved the relative importance of chemical manufacture and fires as sources of dioxin. We do not know the amount of dioxin that has been produced as an industrial by-product, how much of that was destroyed, or how much of it was dispersed in the environment and protected from degradation. Neither do we know how much is produced by fire.

Moving ahead from the observation that dioxin is not ubiquitous in the environment, we can conclude that our own societal activities, especially manufacturing chemicals, produced some major part of it. Since trichlorophenol is no longer manufactured in the United States, that source holds no importance for the future. Moreover, no more still bottoms will be cleaned out and used to suppress dust. Herbicides made from trichlorophenol will not be formulated and sprayed. Those are all problems of the past. Dioxin, already present in the environment, may require cleaning up so as not to expose people, but less dioxin produced as a by-product of chemical manufacturing will be added to the environment. Thankfully, the problems of dioxin derived from manufacturing will never grow larger. That changes, for the better, the problems we face, reducing the amount of effort that should be necessary to control exposure. Yet, dioxin still exists, and wherever it comes from, society is concerned about its potential impact on humans.

CHAPTER 3

AGENT ORANGE AND VIETNAM

More than any other issue or controversy, Agent Orange keeps the topic of dioxin alive and in the public's attention. It is impossible to do more than speculate what the dioxin issue would be if the Vietnam War had been different, but it is entirely possible that Agent Orange might be a forgotten issue, and dioxin a smaller problem.

Despite its profoundly divisive effects on our country, the Vietnam War is defined only by murky margins. It was not a declared war; starting out as an aid mission to supply arms and advice, it escalated. Nor did the United States invade Cambodia; it carried out an incursion. The end in Southeast Asia was neither victory nor rout; it was a winding down.

The United States, its people deeply divided over the advisability and conduct of the war, showed little appreciation for the soldiers' courage and endurance. The departure of thousands of young men and women who entered the armed services, trained, and flew to "Nam" for a year went unnoticed except by families and friends. Their return, 58,000 in body bags but the majority alive, attracted little more attention.

Instead, in many minds, the Vietnam War servicemen ceased being individuals and became personifications of the country's war-making policy. Everyone who watched television during those years knows that the United States military machine produced wholesale death and destruction. Appalled by the magnitude of the killing, citizens opposed to the war directed part of their outrage at the veterans who had served as volunteers or draftees. Veterans, returning to the United States and relieved to have survived, were greeted with "baby killer" and worse epithets from war protesters.

Many Vietnam veterans perceived themselves and continue to perceive themselves as undervalued and ignored by the country that sent them to war. Enlisted or drafted, many entered the service with few marketable skills. More than ever before, they went in right out of high school, and the average age of infantrymen was lower in the Vietnam war than in any other. The military trained and equipped them for war, but for few other occupations. When they returned, the two years in the armed services provided only a few with a leg up in the rapidly changing civilian society; many more were left further behind in competition with those who had not served.

They returned to a country that granted no heros and no parades. Rather, the reception was cold at best. To some extent, both hawks and doves blamed the veterans for the failed effort in Vietnam. Hawks found it difficult to understand how we "lost" to a third- or fourth-rate power. Doves could not excuse veterans for responding to the country's call and carrying out orders that they denounced as anathema to the country's soul.

Now, over a decade after the last American left Saigon, the country continues to sort out its feelings about the Vietnam war and its veterans. To a marked extent, dissatisfaction and disgust with the war are now directed at impersonal targets—national policy and shortsightedness. The country is apparently moving to a position where it sees its veterans as citizens who served as they were ordered to in an unpopular war, and who served probably no better and no worse than generations of Americans before.

The veterans' lot has improved, a little, insofar as serving in Vietnam is no longer seen as a shameful experience, but improvement has come slowly in a series of compromises and understandings. The saga of the Vietnam Memorial on Washington's Mall provides a microcosm of the deep feelings engendered by the war and the treatment of veterans. The memorial design, selected in a national competition, came from a Yale architectural student, Maya Ying Lin. Her instructor had not thought much of it; he gave her design a B. We don't know what grade he would have awarded his own design that he had entered in the competition.

Most often described as "stark," the monument is a long, shallow V of dark marble laid on its side slightly below ground level. A concrete walk descends to its base, and the viewer's eye sees no adornment on the polished black surface, only a listing of every serviceman and woman known to have died in Vietnam or still classified as missing. Unlike many war memorials, it offers no praise to the war or the people who managed it; intended solely as a monument to suffering and loss, it achieves its purpose.[1]

Some citizens were offended, even outraged, by the monument's design and insisted on adding a more conventional memorial. That addition, a sculpture of three infantrymen, faces the "wall" from about a hundred feet away. The two very different memorials complement and enhance each other; veterans were quick to point out that the three sculptured soldiers appear to be "looking for their names."

Washington natives, like natives everywhere, spend part of their time watching tourists. The most casual observer of visitors at the Vietnam Memorial sees that it evokes strong feelings; it means something. Some visitors apparently search for the name of a dead relative or friend, others simply touch names, at random, overcome by the enormity of 58,0007 dead and missing. The average age at the time of their deaths was 19.

The feuds and disagreements are fading. The polarizing war is passing into the hands of novelists and historians, who will rewrite it as they see fit, but the monument keeps alive appreciation of the service and sacrifice of the men and women who went to Vietnam.

Some soldiers returning from Vietnam bore physical and mental wounds, the inevitable consequence of war. Some worsened and died, others "vegged out," unable to overcome what they had seen, done, or endured. In some cases, there was a direct connection between an event in Vietnam and illness; in other cases, the connection was obscure.

"Unusual" diseases, such as cancer in a young man or woman, spur more inquiries into their cause than the same diseases in elderly people. About 2.8 million Americans served in Vietnam, and in a population that large, relatively rare diseases occur with a detectable frequency. A singular event brought national attention to claims of some Vietnam veterans that Agent Orange was making them sick and killing them. As F. A. Wilcox reports in his book *Waiting for an Army To Die:*

> In the spring of 1978, a twenty-eight-year old Vietnam veteran who appeared on the *Today* show shocked many of the program's viewers by announcing: "I died in Vietnam, but I didn't even know it." As a helicopter crew chief responsible for transporting supplies . . . Paul Reutershan flew almost daily through clouds of herbicide. . . . On December 14, 1978, Reutershan succumbed to the cancer that had destroyed much of his colon, liver, and abdomen.
>
> In the months before he died, Reutershan founded Agent Orange Victims International, and spent all of his waning energies trying to inform the American people about his belief that his cancer was the result of his exposure to a herbicide called Agent Orange.[2]

Following the death of Paul Reutershan, his good friend Frank McCarthy, who had founded an organization directed at obtaining better treatment from the Veterans Administration (VA) for veterans wounded in Vietnam, pressured Victor Yannacone, a Long Island lawyer, to take over the lawsuit that Reutershan had initiated against the Dow Chemical Company, a manufacturer of Agent Orange. McCarthy has continued as a director of Agent Orange Victims International, seeking public recognition of the harm that its members see as having been triggered by Agent Orange.

Both Reutershan and McCarthy had been rebuffed by the VA when they demanded better treatment for themselves and their comrades, and both were disgusted with what they perceived as evasive answers when they asked about the effects of Agent Orange on people. It is entirely possible, had their sacrifices been respected or had the VA and its employees been more responsive, that Agent Orange would not have become a rallying cry for Vietnam veterans who objected to the indifference and even hostility shown them by their country.

Nevertheless, Agent Orange looked like a likely culprit for at least some of the poorly understood health effects striking Vietnam veterans. The military had stopped use of Agent Orange when laboratory tests had shown that its dioxin component caused birth defects in mice. Moreover, that discovery was made at the same time that toxic substances in general attracted widespread attention. In the early and mid-1970s, the country became aware of the pervasiveness of chemicals in our society, and the idea that some diseases, especially cancer, could be caused by chemicals, especially chemicals in the "environment," took hold. The general perception of environmental chemicals as a cause of cancer undergirded the specific claims that dioxin in Agent Orange was causing cancer and perhaps other diseases in veterans.

Possible human health effects were not uppermost in the minds of military men who decided to use herbicides to destroy forests. They were guided by military realities. That jungles and forests are treacherous battlefields, especially for conventional armies fighting against guerrillas, was an early lesson for the United States military. In the French and Indian War, before the American Revolution, George Washington commanded the Virginia component of the British General Braddock's troops that marched on the French Fort Duquesne (later renamed Pittsburgh). Braddock, schooled in European warfare, insisted that a train of supply wagons and artillery accompany his forces on their advance from Fort Cumberland, Virginia. Hacking the 132-mile-long road through the virgin forest consumed 32 days, but it seemed splendid at the time. S. E. Morrison writes in the *Oxford History of the American People:*

> George Washington, late in life, said that it was the most beautiful spectacle he had ever seen. Scarlet-coated regulars and blue-coated Virginians in columns of four, mounted officers and light cavalry, horse-drawn artillery and wagons, and dozens of packhorses, splashed through the rippling shallows [of the Monongahela River] under a brilliant summer sun into the green-clothed forest.[3]

The army rode to disaster, however. Using forested ravines as cover, a mixed force of French regulars, French Canadian militia, and Indians fell upon the British force after it forded the river. The battle ended with two thirds of the 1500-man British force killed or wounded and Braddock dying of wounds. The loss pushed back the British frontier hundreds of miles in North America. Fort Cumberland was abandoned. The British forces moved to winter quarters in Philadelphia before the summer was half over, leaving the Pennsylvania–Maryland–Virginia frontier open to Indian attacks.

Americans quickly learned to use forests to their advantage. A few years later, the Continental Army of the American Revolution exploited forests to overcome the British Army of General ("Gentleman Johnny") Burgoyne that invaded the Colonies from Canada. Felling trees across Burgoyne's forest route slowed his advance to a mile a day, and Colonial forces inflicted two severe beatings on the British.

More recent American military history includes bloody chapters in such forests as Belleau Wood as well as jungles at Guadalcanal and in New Guinea. Those fierce jungle battles were fresh in Americans' memories when the U.S. Army first tested aerial spraying of herbicides in 1944 and 1945. As herbicides were developed for use in agriculture and forestry, the military tested them for the purpose of defoliating forests and jungles and persevered in finding better methods to spray them from aircraft.

Post-World War II conflicts have often pitted conventional vs. unconventional forces. When America went to war in Vietnam, its conventional army fought infantry unencumbered by heavy weapons and independent of long supply lines. Since the American way of war relies on overwhelming firepower to devastate the enemy and hold down American casualties, the jungles of Vietnam hampered the American war machine. Heavy weapons, virtually immobilized in the jungles, were restricted to travel on highways and deployment in large base camps. Our infantry, which required large amounts of supplies, could not use the jungle as effectively as the enemy. In many respects, the battlefield favored the enemy, affording him cover and concealment. It takes only simple logic to figure out that if the battlefield conveys an advantage to the enemy, change the battlefield.

The land war in Vietnam raged across much of South Vietnam, and changing a battlefield of that size is no small task. Yet the United States tried. According to a number of estimates,[4] the Air Force sprayed herbicides on one tenth of the land mass of South Vietnam, about 6600 square miles. In terms of United States geography, that area is roughly the same as the land area of Rhode Island and Connecticut combined. It was an audacious effort, made possible by the United States having airplanes specifically for spraying herbicides and unchallenged mastery of the air. The Air Force dubbed its defoliation activities in Vietnam "Operation Ranch Hand."

The Air Force selected a standard, widely used cargo plane, the two-engine C-123, to spray herbicides (and insecticides). A 1000-gallon chemical tank was carried in the cargo bay, and an enlisted man was seated near the center of the aircraft, controlling the release of chemical spray from spray booms under each wing and the tail of the aircraft, which is shown in the photograph below. The other two crew members were the pilot and co-pilot/navigator, both officers, who were seated in the cockpit near the front of the plane.

In some respects, Ranch Hand missions resembled civilian crop-dusting flights. Both require nerve-wracking flying very close to the ground or tree tops. They differ in that C-123s are heavier and less maneuverable than civilian crop-dusting aircraft; a more obvious difference is that enemy troops fired at the C-123s.

Operation Ranch Hand was the most highly decorated Air Force unit in Vietnam. The bulk of the medals were Purple Hearts, which are awarded to servicemen who are wounded by enemy action: Essentially all their wounds were inflicted by bullets fired from small-caliber ground weapons, rifles and machine guns. To reduce their vulnerability to ground fire, Ranch Hands flew early in the morning, flying down out of the sun in such a way as to interfere with the enemy's aim. That tactic helped, but Ranch Hand planes still continued to take hits, and in the later

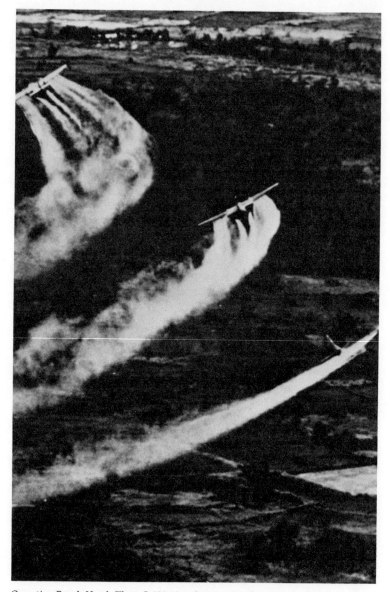

Operation Ranch Hand. Three C-123 aircraft spray Agent Orange in Vietnam. Source: U.S. Government photograph from Alvin Young.

years of Operation Ranch Hand, F-4 fighter planes (Phantoms) strafed the jungle in front of the C-123s to deter ground fire. The strafing missions required close coordination between the Air Force and ground troops to assure that the fighter planes did not strafe our own men. Therefore, two days' notice was given by the Air Force to United States ground troop commanders to be certain that friendly troops were not in the path of the spray missions or that of the accompanying fighter planes.

During the peak spraying years, 1967 through 1969, 24 C-123s were assigned to Operation Ranch Hand. They often flew more than one mission a day, but Agent Orange flights were normally flown only in early morning. Spray missions could involve as many as six aircraft flying abreast at 150 feet altitude and at 130 knots (about 150 miles per hour). Under usual conditions of straight and level flight for the 3½ to 4 minutes necessary to release the herbicide, the spray from each plane covered a swath about 260 feet wide and about 8.7 miles long. The early morning flights, which offered some protection against ground fire, also favored even distribution and deposition of herbicide on the foliage. The planes flew on days with very light winds and arrived at their targets before the land surface had been warmed by the sun.

The many stories of ground troops being drenched with Agent Orange or other herbicides have to be weighed against the fact that the spray rate was three gallons per acre. Furthermore, the majority of Ranch Hand missions were flown over jungles, and much of the spray should have been caught on the tree leaves. Although there are some recorded instances of the entire 1000-gallon load being dumped in an emergency, those "aborts" accounted for less than 1% of all Ranch Hand missions.

Agent Orange emerged as the herbicide best suited for defoliating heavily forested areas. By 1965, it replaced earlier-used herbicides, Agents Green, Pink, and Purple, and between 10 and 12 million gallons of Agent Orange were eventually sprayed in Vietnam, about 60% of all herbicides used there.

Agent Orange was shipped to Vietnam in 55-gallon drums, each marked by an orange-colored band, to distinguish it from other herbicides designated by other color codes. Agent Orange was a mixture of equal parts of the herbicides 2,4-D and 2,4,5-T. Because 2,4,5-T is manufactured from trichlorophenol, which always contains traces of dioxin, all Agent Orange contained small amounts of dioxin.

Both 2,4-D and 2,4,5-T, as well as picloram, which was also used in Vietnam, belong to a class of chemicals known as "plant growth regulators." The exact way in which they cause defoliation is unknown, but in a general sense, the foliage "grows itself to death." The inappropriate growth stimulation causes mismatches among plant parts, so that the vessels that carry nutrients and manufactured products cannot function properly. Its effect is similar to what would happen to an automobile if random parts grew several inches, distorting original proportions.

Some publications refer to "Herbicide Orange" rather than "Agent Orange." That is the residual from a public relations ploy; the Air Force decided that the word "agent" was sinister, suggesting some evil force, and that "herbicide" would be more calming. Unfortunately for that effort, presidents persisted in calling it "Agent Orange," and when President Reagan changed the impossible-to-remember name "White House Interagency Work Group on the Possible Long Term Effects of Phenoxyacetic Herbicides and Contaminants" to the far simpler "Agent Orange Working Group," "Herbicide Orange" was tossed out.

The Air Force sprayed about 90% of all Agent Orange on jungles. Complete elimination of jungle cover required two or three separate missions at two-week intervals to defoliate the three layers of trees present in the jungles. Then, up to three months had to elapse between the spray missions and the complete falling of leaves. As shown in the photograph below, Agent Orange did its job well; leaves did not regrow until 4 to 12 months or more had passed.[5] About 8% of Agent Orange was used against enemy food crops, such as beans, peanuts, potatoes, and mangos.[6]

About 2% of Agent Orange was used by other branches of the military for special purposes. Perhaps most important in terms of human exposure was regular herbicide use around the perimeters of military bases to maintain clear fields of fire and to deny cover to attacking enemy troops. Soldiers, operating back-

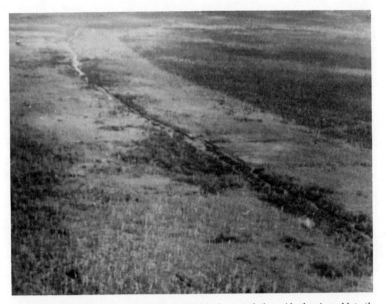

Defoliation, Vietnam. Operation Ranch Hand had sprayed alongside the river. Note the relatively sharp demarcation between sprayed and unsprayed areas. Source: Alvin Young, who obtained it from Capt. Jon Arvik, USAF.

pack sprayers or "buffalo turbine" sprayers from trucks, did the perimeter spraying. Furthermore, Air Force, Army, and Marine helicopters sprayed the same perimeter areas and other well-defined small areas. The Navy sprayed herbicides along the banks of rivers that were used for transportation to keep the foliage down, and again to deprive the enemy of cover. All these uses potentially exposed United States forces to dioxin from drifting herbicides. The ground troops who sprayed it were not generally trained for that job and were probably exposed to high levels from spills and leaks, but they sprayed only rarely and probably were not exposed to as much dioxin as Ranch Hands who serviced planes and flew missions daily.

There is general agreement that defoliation with herbicides

was successful as a military tactic. The Vietcong and North Vietnamese, skillful at traveling through the jungle and using its
cover, were robbed of a vital advantage. Many American lives
were probably saved through this strategy, though of course the
effect in terms of saving lives is unmeasurable.

However, from the very beginning, Operation Ranch Hand
was politically sensitive. The United States government worried
that herbicide spraying would be construed as chemical warfare
and condemned by the international community. As it turned
out, those concerns were not unfounded; late in the war, the
North Vietnamese government adopted that argument. Evidently, the enemy publicized the possible health effects of herbicides. According to Wilcox's book, United States forces countered those claims by using loudspeakers to inform Vietnamese
civilians that the herbicides were not the cause of diseases or
birth defects.[7]

To reduce criticism directed against the United States, standard operating procedures required that the South Vietnamese
government request all herbicide missions. In practice, spray
targets were recommended by United States field commanders
and then passed through the chain of South Vietnamese request
and United States approval. The attempt to identify herbicide
spraying with the Vietnamese, through the request procedure,
was unsuccessful, and spraying continues to be viewed as an
American program.

On the home front, American scientists were leaders in
efforts to stop herbicide use. There is no way to measure how
much of that activity was influenced or motivated by general
opposition to the Vietnam War, a position that is often equated
with liberal political positions. However, in the end, the National Academy of Sciences, which is near the political center,
also described widespread and long-lasting environmental
damage in Vietnam and left open questions about whether or
not human health had been directly damaged by Agent Orange
and other herbicides.

In 1964, a year before widespread Agent Orange spraying
began, the Federation of American Scientists charged that the
United States was experimenting in biological and chemical war-

fare and possibly causing long-term environmental damage to Vietnam. The American Association for the Advancement of Science (AAAS), the largest professional association of American scientists, formally expressed reservations about herbicide use in 1966, when it passed a resolution that recognized that man's use of chemical and biological agents could alter the environment, which in turn could have major, long-term effects on man and the biological systems on which man depends. In 1967, the AAAS urged the Department of Defense to study the long-range effects of herbicides in Vietnam. That same year, more than 5000 scientists signed a petition protesting continued herbicide use as a dangerous precedent for further involvement in chemical and biological warfare. The petition, which was presented to the president's science advisor, and the AAAS protest focused on crop destruction as a barbarous practice that indiscriminately destroyed food of both enemies and allies alike.

The Department of Defense responded to the scientists' concerns by contracting with the Midwest Research Institute (MRI) to conduct a study. The study was limited. No field studies or trips to Vietnam were made; instead, the MRI reviewed 1500 scientific papers and talked with 140 experts in three months. The MRI report concluded that, in general, there was no reason to be concerned about long-term effects. Later, detractors would point out that the MRI had not sought information related to long-term effects. It was not that long-term effects had been looked for and not found; it was that no one had looked. The MRI did draw attention to possible effects from Agent Blue, noting that little was known about the fate of the arsenic in that compound.

In 1968, United States ambassador to Vietnam Ellsworth Bunker ordered a full policy review of the herbicide program. As part of that review, a botanist from the U.S. Agricultural Research Service, Dr. Fred S. Tschirley, toured Vietnam for a short period in early 1968. He pointed out that the mangrove forests on the coasts had suffered more damage than the upland forests. While he found substantial defoliation and some tree killing in the upland forests, it was not the total denuding and near-total killing of trees seen in the mangrove areas. Mangroves are important economically and ecologically as breeding grounds for fish and as habitats for birds and other animals. In 1969, two American zoologists, E. W. Pfeiffer of the University of Montana and Gordon H. Orians of the University of Washington, using private funds, visited the upland and mangrove areas, confirming Tschirley's observations. Professor Pfeiffer had been active in the AAAS discussion of herbicides, and he undertook his trip not only to see firsthand what was happening in Vietnam but also to demonstrate that field studies could be carried out there even as the war continued.

Agent Orange use ended in 1970. The single most important cause was the 1969 release of a report stating that 2,4,5-T caused birth defects in laboratory mice. Acting on that report, the U.S. Department of Agriculture (USDA), which regulated uses of pesticides before the creation of the Environmental Protection Agency, imposed strict regulations on the uses of 2,4,5-T around homes. The report and the USDA's action added credence to the idea that dioxin could cause human health effects, and following on those events, Agent Orange use was suspended in a series of steps, half-steps, and corrections. In October 1969, President Nixon's science adviser announced that Agent Orange spraying would be restricted to "areas remote from the population."[8] That decision appeared to have no importance at all: The Department of Defense (DOD) promptly responded that it did not need to make any changes to comply with that policy. According to the DOD, all spraying had always been done away from populated areas. Five months later, in March 1970, for whatever reasons, perhaps increasing political pressure, the DOD announced that it would reduce herbicide spraying by 25%. But events moved quickly then, overcoming any plans of the DOD to move to other intermediate fallback positions. Senator Philip Hart of Michigan held a hearing on April 1970 during which it was announced that "very clean" 2,4,5-T containing only ⅟₃₀th the concentration of dioxin of earlier-tested 2,4,5-T caused birth defects in laboratory animals. A week later, the DOD made the announcement that it was suspending all Agent Orange use in Vietnam.

Because of these political developments, Agent Orange was

being phased out when the AAAS sent its Herbicide Assessment Committee (HAC), led by Professor Matthew Meselson, to Vietnam in 1970. Scientists, when talking about each other, award few accolades; "He's bright" is effusive praise. Meselson is bright. Over a decade before his trip to Vietnam, he and another young scientist, Frank Stahl, had designed and carried out an elegant experiment that solved one of the riddles of DNA replication. The "Meselson–Stahl experiment" belongs among the tiny number of studies instantly recognizable by the name of the people who designed them.

Meselson had a long-standing interest in chemical and biological warfare, and he was already on record as one of the organizers of the 1966 petition opposed to the use of herbicides in Vietnam. Despite his having taken that position, the AAAS selected him to lead the team of four HAC scientists because of his reputation as being objective and careful. The team arrived in Vietnam in August 1970 and generally confirmed observations made earlier by Drs. Tschirley, Orians, and Pfeiffer about ecological damage. Their report, prepared in time for presentation to the annual meeting of the AAAS in December 1970, also addressed human health concerns. It mentioned the well-publicized vague reports made to them of increased rates of stillbirths and birth defects among Vietnamese living in heavily sprayed areas, and it described the HAC's own efforts to collect reliable information on the rates of defects and stillbirths. However, the obvious war-related problems of record-keeping and data collection prevented them from reaching any definite conclusions.[9]

Concerns about the effects of herbicides in Vietnam spurred Congress to direct the Secretary of Defense to contract with the National Academy of Sciences (NAS) for a study. The contract was signed in 1970 between the time of the HAC's visit to Vietnam and the presentation of their report. Several members of the 17-member NAS committee visited areas of South Vietnam, and the committee examined thousands of photographs of herbicide-sprayed areas to estimate the amount of destruction. Just as the HAC had done, the NAS committee commented on the persistent reports of health effects of herbicides and reported the same lack of firm information. They could find no records to support the claims, but attached great significance to the verbal statements of Vietnamese who lived in the highlands, the Montagnards, that animals and children had been killed by sprays. As an example of the often conflicting assessments of how the war was going in the early 1970s, the DOD had informed members of the NAS committee before they left for South Vietnam that much of the country was secure and that committee members would be permitted to carry out field studies. However, the DOD declared the highlands off limits because of danger from the enemy, so the NAS could obtain no new information about the Montagnards. Similarly, the upland forests or jungles of Vietnam were also labeled off limits, so the NAS committee could not inspect them either.

In summary, the NAS report[10] confirmed extensive damage to the mangrove forests and jungles of Vietnam. Yet the committee's estimate of damage to the upland forests was lower than that made by other groups. Moreover, the president of the National Academy reported bitter quarrels among committee members and reviewers about that estimate. I cannot leave the NAS report without quoting from it concerning the widespread destruction of the mangroves and the future economic loss it means:

> The dead mangroves are being harvested for fuel now, as in the past, although this occupation supports fewer individuals today than before the war. The economic loss, therefore, will be sustained in the future, when the forest has been stripped, unless a vigorous replanting program is undertaken. If this is not done, mankind will have been guilty of a large and ugly depredation of our natural heritage.[11]

The use of "mankind" in the last sentence appears disingenuous. Whatever our country did or did not do during the Vietnam war, we were the ones guilty of "a large and ugly depredation." Two years after publication of the NAS report, President Ford declared that the United States renounced the first use of herbicides in any subsequent war.

Thus, the investigations in Vietnam had confirmed that the

herbicides worked as planned. They killed trees and crops. The same investigations left possible health effects an unanswered question. Though stillbirths and birth defects were reported by Vietnamese both friendly and unfriendly to the United States,[12] records to verify the reports were not available, and wartime conditions prevented conducting studies to investigate the reports.

Since the war's conclusion, there has been little debate about environmental damage to Vietnam. The damage was done, and most people's attitude is that it is now the problem of the Vietnamese. Now concerns are being directed closer to home, to American veterans who cite Agent Orange as the cause of sickness and death among them. Because Operation Ranch Hand dispensed nearly all the herbicides and covered by far the most ground, its activities have been the center of attention. Operation Ranch Hand was also most visible in carrying out herbicide spraying; it was an identified military unit with its own special equipment. Most scientists would agree that the air crews of Operation Ranch Hand—pilots, copilots, and spray operators—and ground crews—men who loaded and serviced the airplanes—were more heavily exposed to Agent Orange (and the other herbicides they used) than any other group. Although the Air Force instructed the ground crews and Vietnamese casual laborers who worked on the bases on methods to minimize exposures to herbicide, few if any precautions were taken to prevent exposure; the mixtures were presumed "safe" by the military. Veterans who sprayed Agent Orange from backpacks, trucks, or boats were also relatively heavily exposed, but because such activities were sporadic and records about who did the spraying nearly nonexistent, it is impossible to verify those exposures.

The core of the bitterness and controversy about Agent Orange, however, does not concern those who sprayed it. Only about 1300 Air Force personnel were assigned to Operation Ranch Hand, and probably a smaller number sprayed it from backpacks, trucks, and boats—all together a tiny fraction of the approximately 2.8 million Americans who served in Vietnam. Instead, the "Agent Orange issue" includes the masses of

ground troops who claim exposures from having been in defoli-
ated areas, having been situated near spray areas, having had
Agent Orange actually sprayed on them and being unable to
wash off the offending stuff, drinking water in which Agent
Orange had collected, and eating fruit from sprayed trees.

I, and most scientists who have considered the exposure
issue, think that it is unlikely that many, if any, ground troops
had accumulated exposures to Agent Orange that even approach those of Ranch Hands or other sprayers. But the veterans who claim damages and their representatives point out
that ground troops, unlike Ranch Hands, did not go to a clean
base, shower, change clothes, eat mess-hall-prepared food, and
sleep in clean beds. The "grunts" remained in the field for days
at a time, stayed dirty, drank whatever water was available,
supplemented their rations with local fruits and vegetables, and
slept wherever they were. Although they might have been exposed to lower concentrations of Agent Orange and dioxin, the
argument remains that they may have been in contact with it for
longer periods.

Another group's social and political lives were changed as
much as, and perhaps more drastically than, those of American
servicemen: the Vietnamese. Agent Orange was not the only
herbicide used against their crops. Agent Blue, an arsenic-con-
taining herbicide, was widely used for destroying rice, against
which Agent Orange is ineffective. Isolating the possible effects
of Agent Orange from those of the other contributors to the total
upheaval of their society appears impossible, yet the Vietnamese, with assistance from members of the international scientific community (including individual Americans), are making
what seem to be earnest attempts to do so.[13]

From small beginnings in 1962, American use of herbicides
increased slightly until 1965, when Agent Orange was introduced, and reached a peak in 1967 through 1969. Almost 75% of
all Agent Orange spraying occurred during those three years,
which were also the peak years of United States participation in
the war. Operation Ranch Hand spraying of Agent Orange ended in 1970 after various investigations of its effects in Vietnam.
There is a general belief that Agent Orange continued to be used

in small quantities around base perimeters for another year. However, the 1.37 million gallons remaining in the Air Force inventory were shipped out of Vietnam in April 1972, and eventually incinerated at sea, thereby ending its military use.

Of course, the end of its military use is not the end of the Agent Orange story. Beginning with some veterans associating Agent Orange with their coming down with cancers, the herbicide now stands accused of causing various diseases in veterans as well as birth defects in their children. Cancer is probably the greatest concern, but liver disease, neurological problems, heart disease, and sexual dysfunction lead a long list that some veterans and their supporters claim to be a result of Agent Orange exposure. Today, a decade and a half after the use of Agent Orange in Vietnam reached its peak, the controversy remains alive in massive epidemiological studies and lawsuits.

CHAPTER 4

WHAT WE KNOW ABOUT AGENT ORANGE AND VETERANS' HEALTH

Veterans who believed that Agent Orange was responsible for their diseases went to the Veterans Administration (VA) asking for care and compensation. In responding, the VA went by the book. Since there was no listing in the book for "Agent Orange diseases," the VA offered the veterans the same medical care available to other veterans, no more and no less, and refused compensation, saying that there was no link between exposures to Agent Orange and disease. Rebuffed by the VA, the veterans did exactly what other citizens do with complaints about executive branch agencies—they took them to Congress.

Congress could have done one of three things. It could have said, "We're sorry about your problems, but there's no such thing as Agent Orange diseases, so you're welcome to seek the usual care that the VA provides to all veterans sick with non-service-connected disabilities, but that ends the government's obligation." It did not do that, however. Neither did it say, "We accept your conclusion that your problems were caused by Agent Orange, and we will provide care and compensation because your problems are related to your service in the Armed Forces." Instead, it took a third course, "We're concerned about your problems, and you may be right that it was caused by Agent Orange. However, before we decide to accept your conclusions, we will have some studies done to investigate your claims."

Why were those studies necessary? Why weren't the veterans' claims accepted at face value? Why was there any disbelief? When Congress first heard the claims, the evidence for the components of Agent Orange, 2,4-D and 2,4,5-T, having caused harm was far from clear. Both had been used for decades in the United States with no convincing evidence of causing disease. Congress's decision that it was therefore reasonable to require evidence draws on a deeply ingrained tenet of American morality and law that people should not receive money in compensation unless they have actually been harmed. To provide compensation without knowing that Agent Orange caused veterans' problems would run against that grain.

Acceptance or rejection of the claims is important because a good deal of money hangs on the decision. If the veterans' diseases are associated with Agent Orange, they are, in the jargon of the VA, "service-connected disabilities," entitling men who suffer from them to compensation. For instance, allegations are commonly made that Agent Orange causes cancer. If every cancer in Vietnam veterans were made compensable, the government would end up paying out a great deal of money. [Assuming Vietnam veterans' cancer rates are the same as the national average, about 25% (700,000) of the 2,800,000 veterans will have some form of cancer during their lives; about 20% (560,000) will die of cancer.] No one, of course, claims that Agent Orange caused every cancer that might arise among the veterans, and a study would also be expected to pinpoint those cancers that it might cause. That information would allow compensation to be made to those who were actually harmed.

Probably of more importance than the money, Congress's eventual acceptance or nonacceptance of veterans' claims will be critical to settling the conflict about whether or not Agent Orange causes disease. Did the government expose its soldiers to a deadly chemical, or have the veterans erred in drawing connections between Agent Orange and disease?

Some people have suggested that the money already spent on studies and earmarked for planned studies would have been better spent if given directly to the veterans. The problem with this suggestion is that the money would not go very far. For instance, the most expensive study will probably cost about $100 million, which under most circumstances is a lot of money. However, were the money to be divided among the many veterans with claims, it would not amount to much. We already know that as a result of the 1984 settlement of a legal suit. In this suit, veterans who claimed damage from Agent Orange sued seven chemical companies that had made the herbicide. The amount of the settlement was $180 million; with interest, the total is now greater than $200 million. Eventually, about 200,000 veterans and dependents joined the suit. If the $200 million were divided evenly, the amount of money per veteran would be about $1000. If $100 million, saved from not doing a study, were made available to veterans and 200,000 veterans asked for compensation from the $100 million, each would receive $500, paltry compensation for a serious disease. A veteran who believes or even has a vague hunch that Agent Orange was responsible for his illness might prefer to see the new studies undertaken. If a study finds convincing evidence for an association between Agent Orange and disease, he can expect at least monetary compensation for his very real suffering.

There are other reasons for wanting the studies to go on. They may provide more information, bringing us closer to the truth about Agent Orange. Perhaps most important is our nation's impatience with not understanding what causes disease. If a person falls ill, we would like to know why. Not only does that satisfy our craving for understanding, it may guide us to preventing similar occurrences in the future.

For most of history, people did not care so much about the causes of disease. Instead, diseases were accepted as a fact of life, unfortunate but unavoidable. It was not until 1861, less than 130 years ago, that a Hungarian physician, Dr. Semmelweis, deduced the cause of "childbed fever." Up to 38% of mothers who delivered in a renowned teaching hospital in Vienna died from the disease. He decided that doctors' hands—still contaminated from autopsies—were the cause of the high death rate. His requiring that doctors wash and rinse their hands in a weak acid solution cut the death rate to less than 1%. When we remember that doctors have treated the sick since the beginning of civilization, it is a surprise that they had not made similar observations and drawn similar conclusions much earlier. Maybe because it forced them to have to reconsider their practices, not all his brother physicians accepted Dr. Simmelweis's discovery. Some ridiculed his ideas. The ridicule certainly contributed to his entering an insane asylum, where he died, perhaps from a beating by his wardens.

Our attitude toward diseases has turned about completely since Dr. Simmelweis's time. We are unwilling to accept any disease as an unavoidable consequence of life. We seek causes for everything. The initial step in the search is that someone—a sick person, family member, or physician—thinks about what might have caused a disease. If those thoughts lead to a suggested association, and if the suggestion appears to have merit, physicians and scientists can go ahead to investigate the putative association.

Paul Reutershan[1] made one of the earliest suggestions that Agent Orange caused serious disease. Extra credence and attention were given the claim that Agent Orange caused his cancer because cancer in a 28-year-old man is unusual, and an unusual disease merits consideration of an unusual cause. If his disease was unique, it might signify that a new and unique cause of disease had been unleashed.

We are all aware that cancer is a far more common killer in old age; deaths from cancer are almost 10 times more frequent in people 65 and older than in younger age groups. Nevertheless, cancer is the number one killer of young adults aged 25 to 45[2] because deaths from infectious diseases, heart diseases and stroke, childbirth, and automobile accidents have been reduced. While deaths from these causes have dropped, cancer death rates have remained relatively constant, accounting for its prominence.

Paul Reutershan died of a cancer in his pelvis that grew so wildly out of control that pathologists could not decide what organ or tissue it had originated from. About 1000 men and about 800 women between the ages of 25 and 29 died from cancer the same year. Therefore, death from cancer at age 28 is uncommon but far from unknown. There has been no trend either upward or downward in death rates from cancers for men 25 to 29 years old since records began to be kept in 1933. Instead, the rate has fluctuated slightly from year to year. If deaths from cancers at those ages had been unknown before the mass production of chemicals began in the early 1940s, or if it had skyrocketed after that date, we could consider a connection between it and modern chemicals. Neither happened. It is clear that young men died of cancer before Agent Orange was used. Whatever caused any one of the other nearly 2000 deaths among young men and women in 1977 could have caused Paul Reutershan's.

Any discussion of cancer causation is complicated by the latent period that separates the time of exposure to a carcinogen from the appearance of the disease. In general, it is accepted that latent periods can be as long as 20 or 30 years. Paul Reutershan died about six years after serving in Vietnam. So little is known about latent periods for various cancers that we cannot dismiss a latent period that short. However, as we will see when we discuss various studies, there is no convincing evidence for excess cancers among Vietnam veterans, further weakening any conclusions that can be drawn from Paul Reutershan's tragedy.

In his 1983 book, Wilcox[3] makes the point that "hundreds" of men with testicular cancer had joined the class action suit against the makers of Agent Orange. Again, hundreds of cancers in young men seem unusual, suggesting that Vietnam veterans are experiencing adverse health events at an unexpectedly high rate. Closer examination reveals nothing unusual in those numbers.

There are about 2.8 million veterans of Vietnam, and the average age of the men who served there was 19.2 years. Unlike other cancers, testicular cancer is most common in young men 20 through 35. I estimate[4] that there will be over 2300 testicular cancers among Vietnam veterans. Therefore, the presence of "hundreds" of men with that cancer in the Agent Orange lawsuit does not mean that veterans are suffering from any unusual or unexpected number of testicular cancers.

Neither should we blindly accept *ad hominem* statements such as "I've never seen another case of this disease in a man of this age" that physicians sometimes make. Given the national rate of 8 cases per 1,000,000 men under 30, what is the chance of a particular physician seeing a case of colon cancer in a man under 30? A single physician would have to examine, on average, a total of 125,000 men under 30 before finding one colon cancer. It is unlikely that any physician in general practice would see even one case and far more unlikely that he would ever see two.

The amount of information that can be developed from case reports and comparisons with national rates is limited. Generally, these shortcomings are overcome by carrying out epidemiological studies that focus on a possible relationship between exposure and diseases.

When veterans began pressing their claims about Agent Orange, the Department of Defense (DOD) insisted that there was no possible association between the herbicide and disease among ground troops because Ranch Hand missions had been flown far away from United States forces. At the same time, the DOD could not deny that the Ranch Hands themselves had been exposed. In the fall of 1978, seven months after Paul Reutershan's dramatic pronouncement on the *Today* show, the Surgeon General of the Air Force promised Congress and the White House to investigate the health of Operation Ranch Hand veterans. The "Ranch Hand study" has merit, since we know the men included in the study were exposed to Agent Orange during shipping, handling, loading the herbicide on aircraft, spray missions, and cleaning of the airplanes and equipment. It nevertheless suffers from the inescapable fact that only 1269 men ever served in Operation Ranch Hand. Therefore, if Agent Orange caused a disease that occurs only very rarely, say less than 1 case in 1300 men, that disease will likely escape detection in the Ranch Hand study. That is a tiny quibble, however. No practical study could detect an event that uncommon. In any case, a study of 1200 men is quite respectable; few epidemiological studies of workers exposed to industrial toxic chemicals have included more than that number. Furthermore, the claims made about Agent Orange point to widespread disease and death, and the Ranch Hand study is large enough to detect big effects—increases in common or even relatively uncommon diseases.

The Ranch Hand study was planned by Air Force scientists and, in keeping with good scientific practice, reviewed by other scientists. The review carried out by the National Research Council of the National Academy of Sciences emphasized that the relatively small number of Ranch Hands would make it impossible to detect diseases that occur only rarely. If the council had expected Agent Orange to double the frequency of cancer or to double the number of deaths at early ages, it would not have included that reservation about the size of the population. The study is big enough to detect a doubling of those events. Nevertheless, the council scientists did not expect to see any such increase in cancer or early deaths because they considered the premise that Agent Orange had caused disease to be very unlikely. So, even before the Ranch Hand study was off the drawing board, there was a clear dichotomy between claims that Agent Orange was the cause of overwhelming disease burdens and the expectations of many scientists that there would be few, if any, detectable effects of exposure. Even though results of the now-completed studies support the scientists' positions, these markedly different perceptions persist to this day.

In epidemiological terms, the Ranch Hand study is a "cohort" design.* By comparing the morbidity (illness) and mortality experiences of the Ranch Hand cohort to another cohort that was unexposed to Agent Orange, scientists plan to tease out which diseases and deaths might be associated with exposure. For comparison, the Air Force selected members of other Air Force units who flew the same kinds of planes as Ranch Hands in Vietnam but who had not sprayed Agent Orange. This is appropriate because Ranch Hands and their "comparisons" had received similar training and had lived under similar conditions in Vietnam.

For each of the Ranch Hands in the study, the Air Force

---

*"Cohort" was originally a military word, describing a tenth of a Roman legion. When used in epidemiology, it refers to a group of people who have shared similar experiences.

selected 5 comparisons.[5] The analysis of the study compares the frequency of disease in the Ranch Hands to the frequency in the controls; including more comparisons makes the study more powerful because it increases the precision of the measurement in the control group. For instance, the certainty that the frequency of a disease is 1% is far greater if it is found 50 times in 5000 people than if it is found 10 times in 1000 people. Knowing the control rate with greater certainty increases the chances of detecting any differences that might be present between Ranch Hands and comparisons.

The Air Force sent letters to the most recent address for each Ranch Hand and comparison. Some letters were returned because the addressees were deceased, and from that and examining Air Force, VA, and Social Security files, the researchers determined which Ranch Hands and comparisons had died. It was then a straightforward matter to obtain death certificates for each of the dead men and to compare the ages at death and causes of death in the two populations. The table below shows the number of Ranch Hands and comparisons who had died as of December 31, 1983.

The most important numbers in the table are in the columns "percentage dead." Among the Ranch Hands and comparisons, both still relatively young men, there have been few deaths. The overall death rate in the two populations is identical, 4.3%. Small differences are seen in comparing subunits of the cohorts. For instance, nonblack Ranch Hand pilots, navigators, flight engineers, and black "other enlisted men" have lower mortality rates than their comparison group counterparts. In contrast, nonblack Ranch Hand "other officers" and "other enlisted men" fared poorer than the comparisons. When the data in the table are subjected to statistical analysis, none of the small differences seen between the Ranch Hands and comparisons is significant.* It is generally agreed that Ranch Hand enlisted men

---

*I will take this opportunity to comment on statistical significance. The percentage of dead nonblack Ranch Hand pilots is 3.4%; that of comparison pilots, 4.3%. While the percentages differ, they are based on such small numbers that the differences could be due to chance. For example, if there were only 3 more

were more exposed to Agent Orange than the officers. The non-flying enlisted men loaded herbicide into the planes and repaired and cleaned the airplanes following missions. The enlisted flight engineers sat near the 1000-gallon herbicide tanks during the spray missions and could have been covered with Agent Orange when tubing or pipes leaked or broke or were punctured by enemy fire. Yet there are no significant differences between the death rates of Ranch Hand and comparison enlisted men. The importance of the control group in interpreting the results is highlighted by the death rate of black flight engineers. As of the end of 1983, 13% of black Ranch Hand flight engineers had died, a larger percentage of deaths than in any other Ranch Hand subgroup. However, that percentage is matched by the rate seen in black comparison flight engineers, indicating that Agent Orange was probably not the cause of excess deaths. The reason for the higher death rates in black flight engineers is not known.

There were some significant differences found when Ranch Hands' death rates were compared to those in other defined populations. For instance, the Ranch Hand officers' mortality rate through the end of 1983 was only 38% of the rate of retired, nondisabled, Air Force officers. This lower rate means that for every 100 deaths in the retired officers, there were only 38 deaths among Ranch Hand officers. This finding makes sense because the retired officer population includes men who "flunked their physicals" and, although not disabled, no longer met the physical requirements for active duty military service. The Ranch Hand population includes men still on active duty, discharged and working at other jobs, and retired. All other things being equal, their mortality rate would be expected to be lower than that of a population of retired officers. The finding of a lower mortality rate in Ranch Hand officers when compared to

---

deaths among Ranch Hand pilots, bringing the total to 15, the percentage of deaths in the two cohorts would be identical. Statistical tests are used to estimate the likelihood that observed differences are "real" and not due to chance. According to those tests, the difference between 3.4 and 4.3% might very well be due to chance, and the best summation of these data is to say that there is no evidence for any real difference.

Death Rates of Ranch Hands and of a Comparison Group of Air Force Personnel Unexposed to Agent Orange[a]

Race	Occupation	Ranch Hands			Comparisons		
		Number of men	Number dead	Percentage dead	Number of men	Number dead	Percentage dead
Nonblack[b]	Pilot[c]	350	12	3.4	1740	74	4.3
	Navigator[c]	82	2	2.4	390	14	3.6
	Other officer	25	1	4.0	123	3	2.4
	Flight engineer[d]	191	7	3.7	935	51	5.5
	Other enlisted man	532	28	5.3	2628	101	3.8
Black	Pilot[c]	6	0	0	13	0	0
	Navigator[c]	2	0	0	10	0	0
	Other officer	1	0	0	2	0	0
	Flight engineer[d]	15	2	13.3	75	10	13.3
	Other enlisted man	52	2	3.8	255	12	4.7
TOTALS:		1256	54	4.3	6171	265	4.3

[a]Source: USAF School of Aerospace Medicine. *Project Ranch Hand II: Mortality Update—1984*. (United States Air Force: Brooks Air Force Base, Texas), February 1985. p. 12.
[b]Includes Caucasian, Asiatic, and Mexican men.
[c]Officer. [d]Enlisted man.

the general male population is also expected because the general population includes men too ill to work and suffering various impairments that increase the likelihood of death.

The frequency of death among Ranch Hand officers is higher than in active duty Air Force officers, also is expected. The active duty officers are examined yearly, and those with less than optimal health must leave the service.

The mortality experience of Ranch Hand enlisted men is better than that of the general United States male population and almost the same as the retired enlisted man population. Neither difference is statistically significant, however. Just as was observed for the officers, Ranch Hand enlisted men had a poorer mortality experience than active duty Air Force personnel. Again, however, the observed difference is not significant.

While overall death rates are of interest, deaths from diseases that might be caused by Agent Orange or dioxin are of more concern. Of these diseases, cancer is the most commonly mentioned. Therefore, the finding that Ranch Hands have no excess cancer is especially significant. The data in the table below show that the death rate from malignant neoplasms (cancers) in Ranch Hands was 68% of the rate seen in the comparison officers and enlisted men.

People who are convinced that Agent Orange causes cancer will not accept this finding as showing that Agent Orange does not cause cancer. Instead, they may suggest that 20–30 years often pass between exposure to a cancer-causing substance and the appearance of the disease. Since heavy spraying of Agent Orange began in 1965, about 18 years had passed between the beginning of heavy spraying and the Air Force's collection of the data shown in the tables. However, additional mortality data are collected and released annually, and if there is an increase in cancer mortality, it will be seen in the years to come.

There are other differences in causes of death between Ranch Hands and comparisons; in particular, the death rate from digestive system diseases was higher in Ranch Hands. This observation will be followed up through yearly updates of the mortality experience of the Ranch Hands and comparisons. For the time being, it is important to note that neither the lower

Comparison of Specific Causes of Death Observed among Ranch Hands
and Comparison Air Force Officers and Enlisted Men[a]

| Cause of death | Number of deaths | | Frequency of deaths (Ranch Hands/ comparisons)[b] |
	In 1256 Ranch Hands	In 6171 comparisons	
Accident	19	94	99%
Suicide	3	16	92%
Homicide	2	4	245%
Parasitic infections	0	4	—
Malignant neoplasms	6	43	68%
Uncertain neoplasms	0	2	—
Endocrine system disorder	1	1	—
Mental disorder	0	1	—
Nervous system disorder	0	2	—
Circulatory disorder	17	75	111%
Respiratory disorder	0	5	—
Digestive system disorder	5	13	189%
Genitourinary disorder	0	3	—
Ill-defined	1	2	—
ALL CAUSES:	54	265	100%

[a]Source: Adapted from USAF School of Aerospace Medicine. 1985. p. 14.
[b]Frequency of death among Ranch Hands divided by frequency in the comparison group, expressed as a percentage.

cancer death rate nor the higher digestive system death rate is statistically significant. Proportionally more Ranch Hands were murdered after returning from Vietnam. However, that could be related to Agent Orange only if some sort of neurological damage caused Ranch Hands to more often behave in such ways as to get themselves into dangerous situations. No other information supports that idea. Also, in the case of homicide deaths, the difference between Ranch Hands and comparisons is not statistically significant. All in all, examination of death rates from particular causes does not suggest that Agent Orange exposure of Ranch Hands is causing increases. (The Air Force had not released the complete update of mortality for calendar year 1984 at the time this book was written, but I had learned that one Ranch Hand and 20 comparisons died during that year. Those deaths bring the totals to 55 and 285 respectively and slightly lower the ratio of Ranch Hand deaths to comparison deaths to 95%. The mortality data from 1984, if considered by themselves, might be construed as indicating that Ranch Hands' mortality is less than the comparisons because the expected ratio of deaths for any year is expected to be 1 : 5, not 1 : 20. A more reasonable conclusion is that the percentage of deaths fluctuates from year to year in the Ranch Hand and comparison populations as would be expected in populations that do not actually differ in mortality. The data are also a reminder to draw only tentative conclusions when data about human morbidity and mortality are collected only over a short period of time, like one year, and when comparisons are based on small numbers.)

As already mentioned, Ranch Hand officers have significantly lower death rates than retired Air Force officers and the general male population; other comparisons show they have lower rates than West Point graduates and civil servants, and higher rates than active duty Air Force officers.[6] If these differences continue, Ranch Hand officers, as a group, will live longer than any of the other groups except the active duty officers. The frequency of mortality seen in Ranch Hand enlisted men is just about the same as that seen in comparable populations. Their death rate is lower than that of the general male population, about the same as that of retired Air Force enlisted men, and higher than that of active duty Air Force enlisted men and civil servants, but none of the differences is statistically significant.[7] Taken together, these statistics show that Ranch Hands are not dying at high rates or at early ages.

Scientifically, the Ranch Hand results are extremely important. *They represent a careful study of the only men known to have been exposed to Agent Orange.* What, if anything, the results mean depends partly on the beliefs people bring to interpreting them. People who believe that Ranch Hands were most exposed to Agent Orange will interpret these data as showing that Agent Orange has not caused excess mortality. Furthermore, accepting that Ranch Hands are most exposed leads to a more general conclusion: Since Agent Orange is not associated with excess deaths in Ranch Hands, it will not be found to be a cause of high death rates or deaths at early ages in any group of veterans.

People who believe that the Ranch Hands were not the population most exposed to Agent Orange view the Air Force results as limited. The results say nothing about the effect of Agent Orange on any other population that might have been more highly exposed.

Were Ranch Hands, in fact, the most exposed population? As an identifiable group, certainly. No group of ground troops was comparably exposed. However, some people, including a few scientists and physicians, argue that the conditions of exposure were so different between Ranch Hands and other servicemen, especially Army and Marine infantry, that studies of Ranch Hands provide no information about ground troops. The basis of this argument is not so much that the infantry was exposed to more Agent Orange as that the conditions of exposure accentuated dioxin's effects.

Ranch Hands slept in clean beds, ate in permanent mess halls, and bathed and changed to clean uniforms after flying missions and servicing aircraft. Infantrymen, as in all wars, were dirty; they stayed in the field for days, sleeping where it was possible, supplementing their rations with what fresh fruits and vegetables they could find, and taking water from available supplies. Infantrymen's exposure to Agent Orange depended on the extent to which it was present in the jungle, on soil, on food, and in water. Once an infantryman got Agent Orange on his skin, it was likely to stay there for days until he returned to a base camp for a shower and clean clothes. On the other side of the coin, there are often questions about whether infantrymen were exposed at all.

Regardless of whether some individuals were more exposed than Ranch Hands, there is no evidence that any other identifiable group of veterans was equally or more heavily exposed. This is not the same thing as saying that there were not some servicemen who were more highly exposed. But because their numbers are bound to be small and the men unidentifiable, they cannot be the basis of a meaningful study.

Australia sent several thousand troops to Vietnam, and that country has examined[8] the mortality experience of veterans of its Vietnam army. Death rates among veterans were substantially lower than death rates in the general population. Overall, the death rate of Vietnam veterans was about 83% of the rate for nonveterans; the comparison was even more favorable for non-Vietnam veterans, about 65% of the civilian rate. While the findings of lower death rates among veterans is reassuring, the more interesting and pertinent comparison found that Vietnam veterans' death rate was only 1.29 times greater than that of non-Vietnam veterans.

However, there was no excess of cancer deaths among Vietnam veterans, and the difference in mortality largely occurred in engineers. Among them, there was a large excess of deaths due to "external causes," including motor vehicle accidents, poisonings, suicides, and homicides. It is highly improbable that those excesses can be related to Agent Orange exposure, although they might somehow be linked to Vietnam service. There were also excesses of deaths from digestive diseases and circulatory diseases, including all types of heart disease, among Vietnam veterans. Although a case could be made that these excesses might be related to Agent Orange, six of the seven digestive disease deaths were alcohol-related. The excesses in circulatory disease may be related to heavy drinking as well as heavy smoking in the Vietnam veterans.

The Australians are at about the same place as Americans in interpreting their veterans' mortality. In 5, 10, 20 years, the trends will be clearer. If there are effects of toxic chemicals, they may yet show up. Currently, the Australian veterans of Vietnam are not in a health crisis. They are not dying at alarming rates, and there is no reason to think that the deaths that have occurred are related to Agent Orange.

The Australian Government appointed a Royal Commission on the Use and Effects of Chemical Agents on Australian Personnel in Vietnam to investigate the veterans' complaints and concerns. The Commission's findings, released in late summer 1985, stated that Australian veterans of Vietnam were healthier than the Australian male population and have lower overall and cancer death rates. In addition, reproductive disorders, birth defects, and neurological damage were not found to be associated with exposure to Agent Orange. The Commission did report that some stress-related conditions could stem from wartime service.

Before leaving the Australian veterans, it is worth noting that until the summer of 1985, the Australian government was much more generous about compensating its Vietnam veterans for conditions they claimed resulted from Agent Orange exposure. In particular, if an Australian veteran claimed that he had been harmed, the government had the onus of proving the claim was not valid, otherwise compensation was paid. That policy has now changed, and the veteran bears the burden of showing that the harm is related to Agent Orange exposure. Therefore, after several years of treating their veterans differently, the United States and Australia are now pursuing the same policy.

A few other studies have examined possible connections between service in Vietnam and cancer. The studies have focused on the group of tumors called soft tissue sarcomas, which affect connective tissue—muscle, bone, etc.—that have been reported to occur at greater than expected frequencies among Swedish lumberjacks who sprayed dioxin-containing herbicides.[9]

No deaths from soft tissue sarcoma were reported in the Ranch Hands or the comparisons. In addition, careful medical examinations of the Ranch Hands found no such tumors, although one was found in a member of the comparison population.

Two additional studies have found no connection. The VA examined its hospital records and found that soft tissue sarcomas occurred at the same rate in Vietnam veterans and in other Vietnam-era veterans.[10] Scientists at the National Cancer Institute and the New York State Department of Health[11] interviewed 281 men (or next of kin of men who had died) who had been diagnosed as having these tumors and compared the occupational, military, smoking, drinking, and family histories of these men to other men of the same age who lived in the same areas of New York State. There was no association between service in Vietnam and soft tissue sarcoma.

In contrast to the negative studies, a study of death certificates in Massachusetts found an excess of soft tissue sarcomas among veterans who went to Vietnam as compared to veterans of the same age who served elsewhere.[12] There was no other excess of cancer deaths reported in the Vietnam veterans; only soft tissue sarcomas, of all tumors, appeared at an elevated rate. The Massachusetts study is a limited study, involving no interviews or examination of hospital records. Such additional information is important because of the difficulties of studying soft tissue sarcomas, which are a grab bag of tumors[13] that affect muscle and other connective tissues. For example, independent review of preserved specimens of seven tumors classified as soft tissue sarcomas found that two had been misclassified.[14] The Massachusetts study, as its authors agree, requires follow-up of hospital records and reexamination of preserved sections of tumors.

Although many caveats can be attached to the results from Massachusetts, the finding does support the arguments of those who see a connection between dioxin and soft tissue sarcomas. Right now, it stands alone as the only evidence for service in Vietnam being associated with an excess of cancer.

As with almost every aspect of Agent Orange and health, there is room for disagreement about soft tissue sarcomas. Overall, according to what is known about the relationship between dioxin and soft tissue sarcomas,[15] and Agent Orange or Vietnam service and soft tissue sarcomas, I do not think the evidence shows a connection, but the Massachusetts results cannot be disregarded. If they are supported in other studies, they will take on added significance.

In addition to examining the mortality experience of the Ranch Hands, the Air Force provided each living Ranch Hand and an equal number of comparisons a medical examination comparable to those given to astronauts. The examinations, first given in 1982, will be repeated at intervals over a 20-year period.[16]

For some health effects, the first report from the morbidity study provides all that we will ever know. For others, more information will become available in later examinations. As an example of a completed measurement, the skin disease chloracne occurs soon after exposure to dioxin. Since there were no cases of chloracne detected in the first examination, we can assume that none will be detected later. Another set of health effects that we will learn no more about are diseases that might have occurred long ago and healed. For instance, no excess of liver disease was detected in Ranch Hands, but more often than the controls, they reported past liver disease. It is likely that if any liver damage was related to Agent Orange, it would have healed in the years since exposure ended, and we probably know as much about possible liver damage now as we ever will. Cancer provides an example of a disease that we expect to learn more about in the future.

On the most subjective measure of health—answers to "How do you feel?"—more Ranch Hands than comparisons rated their own health as fair or poor. One possible explanation for their self-perceived poorer health is that they considered it to have been affected by Agent Orange. A person who believes he is at higher risk may suffer health consequences, as was found among people who were near the Three Mile Island nuclear accident and who more often reported stress-related conditions. Certainly, the Ranch Hands know that they have been exposed to Agent Orange, and that knowledge may cause some to worry more about their health. In addition, Ranch Hands' perceptions of poorer health may be based on past disease. The Ranch Hand group more often reported that they had suffered from psychological, liver, and kidney diseases since returning from Vietnam. Even this observation may be skewed, because Ranch Hands, more concerned about their health, might do a better job of recalling past diseases. That possibility could be investigated by examining physician and hospital records. However, all the records of the more than 2500 men who were examined would have to be collected, and differences among individual physicians and hospitals in record-keeping would greatly complicate interpretation. More important, the continual collection of information as part of the Ranch Hand study will provide more definitive measurements.

There was no evidence for excess cancer or heart disease among Ranch Hands and no soft tissue sarcomas. The cancer finding of most interest was an excess of nonmelanoma skin cancers in the Ranch Hand group. These cancers are not generally life-threatening and are thought to be caused by exposure to ultraviolet radiation in sunlight. The investigators plan to gather additional information about exposure to sunlight to assess this finding.

The results of heart and circulatory system examinations revealed few differences and none of significance. Although Ranch Hands more often had poorer pulses in their feet, this finding is not known to correlate with any disease; it was more common in men who smoked, and no one has an explanation of how it can be related to exposure to dioxin. Ranch Hands over 40 years of age who smoked manifested heart disease more often than did the over-40 members of the comparison group who smoked. The report does not attempt to explain the findings, but the investigators state, "Future reports will explore a theoretical synergism [interaction] between cigarette smoking and herbicide exposure."

Other differences were found on psychological interviews and tests. Although high-school-educated Ranch Hands did as well as high-school-educated comparisons on tests for central nervous system functioning and intelligence, the former, by a small margin, more often reported past emotional or psychological illness and neuropsychiatric symptoms and complaints after their return from Vietnam. They also did less well on assessments of behavior and personality. In contrast, no differences were seen between Ranch Hand officers and comparison officers.

The differences in emotional and psychological measures can be made to fit into a hypothesis that Agent Orange causes psychological problems. Although the correlation is not exact, high-school-educated Air Force personnel are almost all enlisted men, and college-educated personnel are generally officers. If

Ranch Hand enlisted men were more exposed to Agent Orange, then the poorer psychological performance of the high-school-educated Ranch Hands might be associated with exposure. The theory's greatest weakness may be that all the differences that were noticed depended on recall and subjective opinions. In any case, the theory will become more solid or disappear with time as the differences between the high-school-educated Ranch Hands and comparisons increase or disappear on reexamination.

Regardless of the reservations that may be attached to the psychological results, this area deserves careful attention. It is one of the few that suggests any difference between Ranch Hands and comparisons. Furthermore, nervous and psychological complaints are common among other veterans who claim harm from Agent Orange.

The first report from the Ranch Hand morbidity study notes only small differences between Ranch Hands and comparisons, many of which have no clinical importance. The Air Force investigators stress that the effects of known risk factors—smoking, age, education—are stronger than are the differences between Ranch Hands and comparisons. For instance, smoking, far more often than service in Operation Ranch Hand, is associated with heart disease. And, of course, heart disease is more common in older men.

The primary reason for gathering information about various known risk factors is to adjust the analyses so that effects are not wrongly attributed to Agent Orange. Without these adjustments, the study results would be of little value. The second reason is that finding known associations—between smoking and increased heart disease and pulmonary problems, for instance—provides evidence that the study design produced reliable results. Had these associations not appeared, doubt could be cast on the results of the Ranch Hand–comparison analyses.

The most consistent and striking findings of the Ranch Hand study are the differences between officers and enlisted men. As of the end of 1983, a smaller proportion of officers (3.8% of Ranch Hands and comparisons combined) than enlisted men (4.5% of Ranch Hands and comparisons combined) had died, and the morbidity study found officers to be healthier on essentially every measure. In general, officers come from higher socio-economic classes than enlisted men. They have, on average, more education and probably more access to health care and good health advice during infancy, childhood, and adolescence, and their mothers probably had better medical care and nutrition during their pregnancies. As a result of these advantages, officers, at least through their early adult years, are healthier than enlisted men. These observations, which have been seen in other studies of military personnel, seem important to us as a nation that seeks to provide everyone an equal opportunity. We might pay more attention to the effect on later life of the quality of life and good health care at young ages.

The Ranch Hand study, like all the investigations of veterans' health, was planned, executed, and reviewed by scientists. Nevertheless, the final use of the study results is not scientific; it is for policy-making. No member of Congress has interpreted the Ranch Hand study as a cause for introducing legislation to compensate veterans. Instead, the results have been somewhat ignored by some people who are convinced that Agent Orange harmed veterans because of the differences in the way Ranch Hands were exposed as compared to infantrymen. While Washington policy makers may have taken little heed of the results, the results are becoming important in how the Agent Orange issue is presented. Specifically, newspaper editorials are a still-powerful voice in shaping public opinion, and the *New York Times*[17] has interpreted the Ranch Hand study as putting to rest most of the claims of harm from Agent Orange:

> The [Ranch Hand] pilots who sprayed the herbicide were exposed to it [dioxin] daily. In their tour of duty they received a thousand times more than would ground troops by being sprayed directly. Yet a survey of the pilots' health [the Ranch Hand study] . . . showed no unusual incidence of diseases. . . .

The studies of veterans' health, such as the Ranch Hand study and the ongoing studies of ground troops, provide information to everyone with an interest in Agent Orange. But that is all they provide—information. The real bottom line in the Agent

Orange controversy is the decisions to be made about whether or not the Federal government should provide care and compensation to veterans who claim they were harmed and whether or not manufacturers of the herbicide should be held liable for damages caused by their product. The most important decision to date is the settlement of the legal suit brought by veterans against manufacturers of Agent Orange.

After his cancer had been diagnosed, Paul Reutershan initiated a suit against the Dow Chemical Company claiming that Agent Orange made by the company had caused his disease. Other veterans, suffering from various diseases or having fathered children with birth defects, either sued or considered suing. After Mr. Reutershan's death, some of his friends persuaded Mr. Victor Yannacome, the Long Island lawyer who had litigated the banning of DDT, to file a suit against Dow and other chemical manufacturers on behalf of Mr. Reutershan, other veterans, their survivors, and their children. The suit, filed in 1979, claimed that dioxin in the Agent Orange used in Vietnam had caused cancer and other serious health effects among veterans and birth defects in their children.

Over five years later, the lawsuit ended in a settlement agreed to by the lawyers of seven chemical companies and the veterans. The settlement was reached over the first weekend in May 1984. Chief Judge Jack B. Weinstein of the United States District Court for the Eastern District of New York, who is convinced that a jury could have heard and understood complicated testimony about Agent Orange's health effects and reached a just decision,[18] planned to begin jury selection on May 7. A few days earlier, he told the lawyers for the veterans and the chemical companies to come to the Federal Courthouse in Brooklyn and to bring their sleeping bags because there was one last chance to hammer out a settlement before the time-consuming and expensive jury trial would begin.

Courthouse rooms were provided for the camps of opposing lawyers, employees of the court shuttled between them with messages, and bargaining sessions were held in the presence of the judge or Kenneth Feinberg, a Washington lawyer who was the special master in the case. In the settlement, while denying that Agent Orange had caused adverse health effects, the companies paid the veterans $180 million.

The settlement was the most expeditious end to the proceedings for both sides. In the long run, the companies saved money, even if they would have eventually won in a trial. The trial itself, followed by appeal after appeal, would have generated enormous legal fees and much negative publicity, and would have kept the companies under a gray cloud of uncertainty about their potential liability. The day after the settlement, Dow's stock went up, illustrating that settling the lawsuit was good for the company. The veterans also probably came out ahead. According to Judge Weinstein, who had read all the evidence introduced into the case,[19] the evidence did not support a finding that Agent Orange had caused disease among the veterans. Assuming that a jury would have reached the same conclusion, the settlement, although a small amount of money if divided among all the veterans who sued, represents more than the veterans would have gotten in a jury trial. And for the veterans also, years of litigation and uncertainty, with ever-mounting obligations to lawyers, was avoided. Of everyone involved, the attorneys are the only group that might have fared worse under the settlement. The judge limited total fees for veterans' lawyers to under $10 million. The first priority was to pay lawyers who had put up their own money ($750,000) to bankroll the case. After that disbursement was made, the judge apportioned the money on the basis of the quality and importance of the work done; the Agent Orange suit was no lawyers' windfall.

The $180 million began earning more than $60,000 daily interest. The next problem was deciding who was to receive the money. About 10,000 veterans were members of the class action suit at the time of the settlement. However, other veterans who claimed harm could join the class afterward. By summer 1984, the court expected a total of about 70,000 in the class, but by early 1985 when the time for enrollment expired, 200,000 veterans had joined the class. Members of the class vary greatly in their claims. Some have cancer, some are widows and orphans, some are "nervous," some lack energy and don't feel well, and some have children with serious birth defects.

Because the companies did not admit that their products had caused any disease and because, in the judge's opinion, there was no proof that Agent Orange had caused the veterans' health problems, the judge did not require that a veteran show a relationship between exposure and sickness. Instead, "compassion—not scientific proof—would be the underlying principle"[20] of distributing money. During the summer and fall of 1984, the judge held hearings in five cities to listen to veterans' opinions about the settlement and the distribution of money. In November, he met with an Advisory Board of veterans to review a number of plans for the money from the settlement.

As plans stood in July 1985, $150 million of the settlement funds will be designated for compensation to veterans who suffer total disability and to the survivors of veterans who have died. It is estimated that about 17,000 veterans will qualify for total disability payments and survivors of about 10,000 will receive death payments before the fund is exhausted. The maximum amount of money to be received by claimants who were totally disabled before January 1985 will be $25,000; those who become disabled after that time will be eligible for a maximum of about $14,000. Death payments will be $5000.[21] The veterans in the fairness hearings insisted that the disability payments exceed the death payments to avoid the impression that a veteran was worth more dead than alive. An additional $45 million will establish the Agent Orange Class Assistance Foundation to provide aid to children, spouses, and veterans ineligible for cash awards. The aid will consist of information and counseling services.

Some people say that the Agent Orange lawsuit decided nothing because the case did not go to trial. In any case, many people see disease causation as a scientific issue, not a legal one. Other people who accept the government's position that the chemical companies were less than honest in presenting their defense[22] would have liked to see the companies punished. For some veterans, the settlement was at least partial victory: "The veterans may not be able to prove that those [serious] illnesses resulted from their exposure; however, no one can prove that they didn't."[23]

In contrast, I think the settlement has a profound and lasting impact on the Agent Orange issue and injected a note of finality into the controversy. The *New York Times* editorial page has been adamant about the lesson from the settlement: ". . . there's no reason to suppose either that veterans were exposed to significant amounts of dioxin in Vietnam, or that they have any symptoms for which dioxin might be the explanation."[24] It quoted from a plan for the distribution of the settlement money, "It is totally uncertain whether any serious adverse health effects could have been caused by the level of Agent Orange exposure veterans might have received in Vietnam."[25] The *Washington Post* has printed similar editorials: "As the federal judge presiding over the settlement has stressed, there is currently no scientific basis for linking any of the diseases claimed by the veterans to Agent Orange exposure."[26] And ". . . there is no solid evidence to support veterans' claims that Agent Orange is responsible for the ailments that they and their offspring—along with many other people in the general population—have suffered."[27]

The effects of the settlement on public opinion will probably be more important than any continuing disagreements among scientists about the nuances of study findings. The court considered those nuances, but the judge's opinion that nothing had been proved, apparently shared by at least some of the veterans' lawyers who agreed to the settlement, was the bottom line.

The lawsuit was brought largely by ground troop veterans. In comparison to Ranch Hands, we know far less about the Agent Orange exposure of these men. That means that any adverse health effects from Agent Orange might be hidden in information collected about groups of ground troops that include both exposed and nonexposed veterans. Only if it is possible to develop a method to estimate exposure to Agent Orange will anyone be able to say something definitive about possible associations between Agent Orange exposure and soft tissue sarcomas or any other health effect among ground troops. To determine the possible effects of Agent Orange on other veterans requires a study that faces up to the problems of determining which veterans were exposed. An immense and expensive study of ground troops who served in Vietnam that will attempt to do that is under way.

CHAPTER 5

WHAT WE MAY LEARN ABOUT AGENT ORANGE AND VETERANS' HEALTH

No one denies that diseases that kill and incapacitate afflict veterans and that birth defects that bring untold grief, pain, and expense strike their children. However, we simply do not know the specific causes of most cancers, most heart attacks, most strokes, most birth defects. Glibly to ascribe veterans' diseases and deaths to Agent Orange is to say that the veterans would have been otherwise free of those calamities. Clearly, that is not possible. On the other hand, to decide that none of the veterans' diseases is related to Agent Orange may seem to go too far. After all, dioxin, which was present in Agent Orange, has at least caused chloracne in occupationally exposed populations.

Regardless of the arguments made by veterans, the executive branch of the government in the late 1970s responded similarly to all claims that Agent Orange had caused disease. It stoutly maintained that ground troops did not enter sprayed areas until four to six weeks after spraying. Therefore, no ground troops could have been exposed by spray missions, for by the time they entered the sprayed area, most of the Agent Orange would have degraded. Moreover, according to the Department of Defense (DOD), it was impossible to track troop movements and match them in any way with Agent Orange spraying.

Those blanket rejections were pushed aside in 1979. In the spring of that year, then-Senator Charles Percy of Illinois requested that the Congress's investigative office, the General Accounting Office (GAO), investigate the possibility that ground troops had been exposed. John Hansen, a GAO employee who was assigned to the Veterans Administration (VA), set out to do what the DOD said was impossible—to compare the location of military units on the ground to the paths of Ranch Hand spray missions as recorded on computer tape. He first attempted to use Army records to locate Army units, but gave up because, in his evaluation, the records were incomplete and poorly kept. He found Marine records in better shape. With the help of his colleagues, he located the positions of several Marine battalions in the northern section of South Vietnam. Despite the DOD's claims that it could not be done, Hansen matched unit locations with spray missions. His report rendered the DOD's denials untenable.

The GAO report[1] showed unequivocally that about 5900 Marines had been within half a kilometer (0.3 mile) of areas sprayed with Agent Orange on the day of spraying. In fact, some units were directly under the path of spray missions. Equally important, the methods used by the GAO demonstrated that the movement of troops, or at least of battalion headquarters, could be tracked over the course of time and their movements and positions compared with the locations and times of Ranch Hand spray missions. Mr. Hansen thinks that one reason the DOD failed to find that ground troops had been exposed was that in 1978 and 1979, the DOD regarded Agent Orange as being of no great concern; the DOD simply did not bother to undertake serious examination of records to investigate veterans' claims. If that impression is correct, DOD employees who judged Agent Orange as being of little importance erred.

Mr. Hansen[2] does not believe that the DOD was covering up when it denied that ground troops had been exposed. Instead, he thinks that the weeks or months that passed between a ground commander's requesting a spray mission and the mission's being flown was partially responsible for the error. During the time between request and mission, troops could be moved into the area to be sprayed, with the men who scheduled the mission being unaware of their presence.

Would Ranch Hand air crews have noticed that they were spraying troops? On spray missions, the planes flew only 150 feet from the ground at about 150 miles an hour and sprayed Agent Orange along an 8-mile path on each mission. From that altitude and at that speed, air crews would have been unlikely to see any troops on the ground in time to stop spraying or turn aside. In any case, when jungles were sprayed, the men in the planes would be unable to see anyone on the ground. Some Ranch Hand spray missions were preceded by strafing fighter planes, which raises the specter that some Americans were exposed to friendly cannon fire as well as to Agent Orange. I am unaware of any reports of Americans being strafed under those conditions, but that could be explained by a number of factors. Most disturbing to think about is that such mistakes were made but that the military has buried references to them. Second, it could be that there were very few fighter-accompanied Ranch Hand missions. Third, when fighters went along with Ranch missions, far greater efforts might have been made to assure that no Americans were in the target area.

The GAO's report recommended that the government "determine whether a study is needed on the health effects of herbicide orange on ground troops identified in our analysis." A month later, in December, Congress passed a law that skipped over the GAO's recommendation to determine *whether* a study was possible. Instead, it directed that the study be done. The law mandates that the VA conduct a study of veterans who "were exposed to any of the class of chemicals known as dioxins" in Vietnam to determine whether there had been any long-term adverse health effects. The law gave the VA six months to plan the study.

Also in December 1979, the executive branch of the Federal government realized that concerns about possible health effects from spraying Agent Orange were problems likely to require major efforts. The surest indication of that realization was the White House's directing the formation of the Agent Orange Working Group (AOWG)[3] to coordinate policy about Agent Orange. As soon as the AOWG met, it was apparent that Agent Orange could not be separated from the problems of dioxin; the two issues were absolutely intertwined, and the AOWG began considering policy about dioxin in general with a special emphasis on Agent Orange. Within a very short time, the Federal government was sponsoring immense amounts of research, and the AOWG spun off a Science Panel to monitor it. There is a general consensus that the AOWG has been instrumental in moving along the Federal research and policy efforts and has made a major contribution to resolving the issues that swirl around Agent Orange and dioxin.

Despite the establishment of the AOWG, years of bickering and indecision among executive branch agencies followed Congress's 1979 order that a study be designed in six months. There was delay after delay in attempting to design a study to resolve whether Agent Orange did, in fact, damage the health of Vietnam veterans. Some delays resulted from scientific problems; in particular, the problem of deciding which veterans had been exposed to Agent Orange bedeviled every attempt to design a study.

Members of the AOWG Science Panel wrestled with the problem of whether or not it was possible to distinguish between veterans who had been exposed to Agent Orange and those who had not. In particular, their discussions grappled with the very real problem of what it meant for troops to have been within a kilometer or two of a spray mission. Did that mean that they had definitely come in contact with the spray? How close to the spray area did troops have to be to be counted as exposed? After much deliberation, the Science Panel decided that there were no simple answers to these questions. Making the matter more complex, its members worried that Agent Orange was not the only chemical to which veterans had been exposed. Other herbicides and insecticides had been widely used, troops had been treated with drugs to prevent malaria, and numbers of soldiers partook of various mind-altering substances commonly available in Vietnam. Was it not possible that any one or some combination of these things might be responsible for any adverse health effects seen in veterans? The Science

Panel decided, despite the GAO's findings, that it really was impossible to separate Agent-Orange-exposed veterans from unexposed veterans and that other exposures should also be considered in any epidemiological study. It proposed that the "Agent Orange study" be dropped and that a "Vietnam experience study" be substituted. The AOWG listened to the Science Panel, and it too decided that a Vietnam experience study made more sense.

Congress responded to the Science Panel's concerns by passing another law that modified the responsibility of the VA. Until that point, the VA had been charged with studying the effects of Agent Orange. The new law said that the head of the VA could expand the scope of the study to include possible long-term adverse health effects from other herbicides, chemicals, medications, or environmental hazards or conditions.

The passage of this law did not still discussions among the Science Panel members about the possibility of a study focusing on Agent Orange. Dr. Jerome Bricker, who, in the 1960s, had worked on the development of the spray apparatus for Operation Ranch Hand, was, in 1981, a civilian employee of the DOD. Sitting on the Science Panel, he proposed a method to estimate whether veterans had been exposed to Agent Orange.[4] Briefly, any body of troops that was within specified distances of a Ranch Hand mission, or within specified distances of an emergency dumping of Agent Orange from a damaged Ranch Hand plane, or in a base camp where the perimeter was sprayed with Agent Orange would be considered exposed to Agent Orange. The number of these "hits" would be summed up for each unit, and those with the most would be assigned to the heavy-exposure category; those with less, to a light-exposure category.

Dr. Bricker's memo also included an estimate of how much Agent Orange would be deposited on a man directly below a spray mission. This kind of calculation is as important to discussions of "exposure" as John Hansen's discovery that troops were under spray missions. If a man was under a Ranch Hand airplane spraying Agent Orange, we know he came into contact with dioxin, but how much? The answer is that we do not know the exact amount that a veteran might have been exposed to, but as can be seen from the calculations in the Appendix, the exposure can be estimated. According to the calculations, no veteran directly under the most dioxin-contaminated Ranch Hand spray was exposed to the minimum dose necessary to cause chloracne. That calculation appears to be correct because fewer than two dozen Vietnam veterans have diagnosed chloracne, and even those cases could have originated from exposure to other chemicals.

It is tricky to try to estimate the amount of dioxin that would enter a soldier's body from chemicals deposited on his clothing. However, a soldier directly under some dioxin-contaminated Agent Orange spraying could receive a dose greater than the amount the Food and Drug Administration estimates to be a virtually safe dose if ingested daily for 70 years. Even 0.5 kilometers away from the spraying, exposure drops to 2% of the maximum; at 1 kilometer, it 0.03%. Other exposures, through ingesting dioxin-contaminated soil or dioxin-contaminated water, were possible, but the amount of dioxin that reached the soil or water would be the same small amount that would have fallen on a soldier. The calculated exposures are thus very low.

So what? Calculations of doses leave many people unconvinced. What if the application rate was sometimes much greater? Or what if soldiers spent many days in contact with sprayed foliage and thereby greatly increased their exposure? What are the possibilities of having been sprayed repeatedly? Maybe there were special risks associated with conditions in Vietnam. For these reasons and considering dioxin's toxicity and the claimed connections between Agent Orange and disease, many people insisted that a study be done. And that was the position that carried the day.

The AOWG considered an epidemiological study that would include three cohorts of veterans—a group of Vietnam veterans classified as exposed, a second group classified as unexposed, and a third group, veterans who had not served in Vietnam. Comparing the health of the three groups would provide information about the effects of Agent Orange and the effects of service in Vietnam.

Before the AOWG had come up with the three-group idea,

the VA had contracted with a group of investigators at the University of California at Los Angeles for a study design. Their plan included only two groups, exposed and unexposed veterans who had served in Vietnam, so it might yield some information about Agent Orange but none about the effects of service in Vietnam as compared to service elsewhere. A third possible study design was to ignore Agent Orange altogether and only compare Vietnam veterans to veterans who served elsewhere. Proposals for study designs and critiques of the proposals continued through 1981 and 1982, and the fact that no study was actually going on was laid at the feet of the VA. In September 1982, both the House of Representatives and the Senate criticized the VA and urged that the VA relinquish direction of the epidemiological studies so that the process would be speeded up. The VA elected to follow this advice; hence, the studies were transferred to the Centers for Disease Control (CDC) in early 1983. The CDC was a good location for the studies because that agency is very strong in epidemiology.

The CDC prepared an outline for the study of Vietnam veterans' health even before the transfer was completed and submitted a full-fledged study plan to the AOWG and the Office of Technology Assessment (OTA) in early 1983. The law that ordered the study of veterans' health to be made had also directed the OTA, where I worked, to review and approve the study plan, and I was placed in charge of the review. Assisted by a 15-member advisory panel including scientists and representatives of companies that had made Agent Orange as well as members of veterans' organizations, the OTA reviewed the CDC plan that was submitted in 1983, suggested some changes, and gave it final approval in February 1984. That was three and a half years after the date Congress had set for the plans to be completed.

The CDC plan describes what is to be probably the most expensive, most complex, and largest group of epidemiological studies ever undertaken. With a budget of $70,000,000, the CDC has had to add about 50 professional staff members to design and carry out the Agent Orange studies during a time that most government agencies are having to cut back personnel. The

CDC resolved the old controversy about whether to do a two- or three-cohort study by proposing a three-cohort study and a two-cohort study; moreover, because of concern about some particular cancers, it added a case–control study.

The aim of the CDC study is to examine three possibilities:

1. that exposure to dioxin present in Agent Orange is associated with adverse health effects among Vietnam veterans—*The Agent Orange Study*.
2. that service in Vietnam is associated with adverse health effects—*The Vietnam Experience Study*.
3. that an elevated risk of developing certain cancers is associated with service in Vietnam and/or exposure to Agent Orange—*The Cancer Study*.

The design of the first two studies is set out in tabular form below.

Results are a long way off: Reports about the effects of

CDC Cohort Studies of the Health of Vietnam Veterans

"Agent Orange Study"			
Cohort[a]	Vietnam service?	Combat?	Agent Orange exposure?
One	Yes	Yes	Yes
Two	Yes	Yes	No
Three	Yes	No	No

"Vietnam Experience Study"			
	Service in:		
Cohort[a]	Vietnam	United States only	United States and Europe	United States and Korea
One	All	None	None	None
Two	None	One third	One third	One third

[a]Each cohort will consist of 6000 Army veterans. All cohort members will be interviewed about their service experiences and health, and 2000 of each cohort will undergo medical and psychological examinations.

Vietnam service on mortality and morbidity are scheduled to be released in 1987; reports about the effects of Agent Orange on mortality and morbidity will follow in 1989 and 1990, about the same time results will be released from the cancer study.

The question of possible effects of Agent Orange will be examined by comparing the health status of three cohorts: combat soldiers likely to have been exposed to Agent Orange, combat soldiers not likely to have been exposed, and noncombat soldiers who were not likely to have been exposed. If combat has had an impact on health, the health experiences of the first and second cohorts should resemble each other and differ from the third. If Agent Orange has had an adverse impact on health, the first cohort's health experience should be different from those of the other two.

The possibility that Vietnam service caused adverse health effects will be examined by comparing the health of a cohort of Vietnam veterans with the health of veterans of service in other areas during the time of the Vietnam war.

All five cohorts are made up entirely of veterans who served one term of duty as enlisted men and who did not advance beyond the rank of sergeant. Each cohort will consist of 6000 men; all the men will answer a detailed telephone questionnaire, and 2000 of each cohort will undergo a thorough medical and psychological examination. By any measure, the CDC study (30,000 questionnaires and 10,000 medical examinations) is a very big study.

The question of whether certain cancers are more common among Vietnam veterans will be examined by a case–control study. Scientists refer to men who have the types of illness being studied as "cases." These "cases" will be identified from cancer registries and records that are maintained by some hospitals and by some city and state health departments across the country. The frequency of Vietnam service among that group will be compared to the frequency among a group of "controls," men who live in the same geographic areas but who do not have the cancers.

Paradoxically, as the CDC's plans for the Agent Orange study have grown more definite, sanguine expectations have faded. The old bugaboo of deciding which veterans are more likely to have been exposed to Agent Orange has come roaring back, borne on unexpected complications. The likelihood of exposure misclassification is staggering and potentially fatal to a meaningful study. As an example of the problems, the CDC, in January 1985, described its latest method for assigning veterans to the exposed category. All members of a battalion who were within two kilometers and three days of a spray mission as measured from the center of the area occupied by the battalion will be considered exposed. The problem is that battalions were spread out over scores of kilometers. Consider that 10 or 100 men in a battalion were actually at the central location, directly in the path of a Ranch Hand mission and covered with spray. Other members of the battalion, some 20 or more kilometers away, would be totally unexposed. But these men would be classified as members of the battalion and called "exposed." At the other extreme, men who were some distance from the central location of their battalion and who were exposed as they passed through an area soon after a spray mission or down a road that had been treated by an unrecorded truck-mounted sprayer could be classified as unexposed. Misclassification from both directions tends to make the two groups—"exposed" and "unexposed"—look more and more alike, a mixture of exposure histories in both. The possibility of discovering any actual differences in health status due to exposure unfortunately decreases with misclassification.

Quite beyond the question of who was exposed are queries about what health effects Agent Orange might have caused and might cause in the future. Arguments about these possibilities have been going on for years and generally proceed down well-marked tracks. Many experts (certainly most, and perhaps almost all) who have considered the very small amounts of dioxin from spray missions are convinced from the absence of long-term health problems (except chloracne) among highly exposed workers that the CDC Agent Orange study will find no health detriment associated with the herbicide. Countering these opinions, veterans claim that the nature of their wartime exposures accentuated the effects of dioxin, and this possibility is a potent argument for doing the Agent Orange study. In response, some scientists point out that veterans do not have the skin disease chloracne, a hallmark of occupational exposure to dioxin, and that absence of that disease is inconsistent with significant dioxin exposure.

This observation, nonetheless, does not end the controversy. There still exists the possibility that exposures to dioxin at levels too low to cause chloracne might cause cancer or other health problems. On scientific grounds, there is no denying this argument; it could be true.

But what we do know about dioxin's health effects runs against the expectation of finding effects from Agent Orange at the levels of exposure experienced in Vietnam. The only health effects for which there is *convincing* evidence from studies of exposed chemical workers are chloracne and some changes in liver and biochemical measurements that so far as we know have no clinical significance and may be the result of other exposures, and there have been inconsistent reports of nerve damage and ulcers.[5] There is no convincing evidence for excess cancer or heart disease in exposed chemical plant workers. The only exception to the statement about no excess cancer in chemical workers is one report about stomach cancers in workers at a German plant. However, no other study of dioxin-exposed chemical workers has found excess stomach cancers, and it is very likely that the stomach cancers in the German workers had a different cause.[6] There are also suggestions that soft tissue sarcomas and perhaps other cancers appeared more frequently than expected in Swedish herbicide sprayers.[7] However, studies in Finland and New Zealand have failed to confirm those results, and the Swedish studies appear less and less convincing. Of course, the CDC would have been remiss if it did not investigate the possibility of soft tissue sarcomas being associated with Agent Orange exposure, and its Cancer Study will provide detailed information about the incidence of these cancers in Vietnam veterans.

Only a fool would deny that combat, killing, seeing friends dismembered, and protracted fear of death would affect survivors' mental health. With that as a given, the Vietnam Experience Study may provide information about specific wartime experiences and subsequent health effects. Still, the power of this study to detect effects is limited. In particular, according to the CDC's own statistical analysis, the Vietnam Experience Study has a good chance of detecting any twofold increases in common diseases such as common allergies and mild respiratory infections. Excesses of rarer diseases will not be detectable unless there is more than a twofold increase in them; the chances of a statistically significant finding decrease with smaller numbers of cases. Psychological problems are probably more common in Vietnam veterans than among many other members of the population, and the Vietnam Experience Study will provide some information about that.

Unfortunately, a study that finds no statistically significant increase does not necessarily mean that there was no effect of Agent Orange or Vietnam service. Instead, the study can only say that Vietnam veterans are not experiencing particular diseases at rates two or more times those seen in other veterans. It is always possible that a still larger study, examining even more veterans, could detect some effects. At the very least, a larger study would reduce the chances of overlooking any effects. However, I cannot imagine that a larger study will be ordered if the CDC studies are negative. If, on the other hand, some effects are found, even at levels below statistical significance, more sharply focused studies can be carried out to investigate the possible connections. The Cancer Study is an example of a focused study.

Unlike the two cohort studies, which are "hypothesis-generating" studies, the Cancer Study is a "hypothesis-testing" study. It has the virtue of asking a specific question: Did Agent Orange exposure or service in Vietnam cause an excess of specific cancers? No results are expected until 1989 or 1990 because that much time is necessary to accumulate a few hundred cases of the rare cancers that are being studied.

As evidence mounts that few veterans were exposed to any significant amounts of dioxin, that veterans probably cannot be divided between those likely and unlikely to have been exposed to Agent Orange, that the Vietnam Experience Study is unlikely to reveal differences in the occurrence of significant health effects, and that the study of selected cancers is less powerful than expected,[8] why does the Federal government move ahead with these expensive and complicated studies? First of all, there is the possibility that there is "something really there." Any possibility that now-undetected disastrous health effects are present among veterans makes it difficult to consider bringing any study to a halt. In response, it can only be argued that there is hardly any reason to think that something is really there. The Ranch Hand study reveals no convincing evidence for health effects from Agent Orange. More important, the Air Force Ranch Hand study will continue for 20 years with periodic reports on the morbidity and mortality of those men. If adverse health effects appear in the Ranch Hands, veterans of the ground forces in Vietnam could be examined for that particular condition or disease.

The Vietnam Experience Study has more justification, but it is investigating even vaguer possible associations. According to the CDC's own calculations, it cannot be expected to detect excesses of anything but the most common of diseases. However, if it comes up negative for medical problems, it should lessen concern that Vietnam veterans' physical health has been seriously harmed. If it is positive and shows some connection between Vietnam service and physical or mental health, it may at least persuade the government to provide more and better health care to veterans.

The Cancer Study seems like a reasonable study. Although VA and National Cancer Institute studies of soft tissue sarcomas show no relationship between service in Vietnam and the occurrence of that tumor, a study of veterans in Massachusetts, as was noted earlier, found an excess among Vietnam veterans as compared to other veterans.[9] Also as mentioned earlier, I do not dismiss the Massachusetts finding, but believe additional work is needed before it can be accepted. The possibility of resolving the controversy about cancer in Vietnam veterans is a strong incentive for going ahead with the Cancer Study. Neither the Agent Orange nor the Vietnam Experience Study will examine enough cancer victims to shed any light on the controversy.

Beyond the technical reasons for going ahead with the studies are political and bureaucratic reasons. Primarily, Congress in 1979 reviewed what was known about Agent Orange and decided that there was not enough information to decide whether veterans had been harmed. Congress then ordered the study, making a promise to veterans that what could be done would be done. Second, of less importance, a strong plan and work force to carry out the study have been secured. The CDC has hired well-qualified people, contracted with independent hospitals and laboratories to gather data, and arranged for the complex mesh of analysis and review necessary to assure the validity of the studies. Of course, overarching everything else are the claims and concerns of veterans who believe strongly that they have been seriously damaged by Agent Orange.

Everyone concerned—veterans, the VA, the CDC, Congress, and the public—wants to resolve the Agent Orange and Vietnam veterans' health issues. The CDC studies are seen as holding out the promise of doing that. However, if more information brings that promise into question—if, for instance, the CDC or the AOWG or the Congress or all of them decide that it is impossible to determine who was exposed and who was not exposed—everyone concerned should be willing to reevaluate the possible usefulness of the study. Being interested in the answers the studies may provide, we should examine the probability of finding answers, and if the probability is low, we should consider not doing the study. Unfortunately, I see little evidence of critical appraisal. Instead, we appear to be going ahead, giving it our best shot without considering that the studies are likely to be inconclusive. I think that no diseases will be found associated with Agent Orange exposure, and if that is the result, we may be little further along than we are right now. Let us assume that the Agent Orange study is negative, that it finds no health effects. Immediately, people who think that result is wrong can say that the exposure classifications are so likely to be off that the study was flawed. And they will be right. Since there is no way to do a better job in classifying exposure, it might be wiser to consider stopping the study. And it might be more responsible to say that exposures were so low that no effects would be expected.

We are in a standoff situation. The CDC studies have a juggernaut quality, rolling along, producing more and more refined plans, with examinations already begun. In November 1984, the CDC placed a $35,900,000 contract with the Lovelace Medical Foundation of Albuquerque, New Mexico, to carry out 10,000 medical and psychological examinations. Beginning June 1, 1985, an average of 334 veterans have been scheduled to arrive in Albuquerque each month for their examinations. This study is thus in progress. In addition, the Research Triangle Institute has a contract to telephone and question 30,000 veterans. Plans have been prepared to examine every bit of information produced by these immense efforts. However, the overriding flaw—that we do not know who was exposed—is being ignored as plans for examination and analysis become more certain and elaborate.

In the absence of any convincing evidence for an "Agent Orange disease," Congress mandated that the VA presume that two diseases—chloracne and a rare metabolic disease, porphyria cutanea tarda—are associated with Agent Orange. The fact that the two diseases are essentially unknown in Vietnam veterans makes the presumption somewhat hollow; few veterans will be compensated. At the same time, Congress's refusal to grant more widespread compensation shows that it is demanding that connections between Agent Orange and other diseases be proved before compensation is given. For that, the studies are terribly important; all possibilities for compensation hang on their results.

Predicting the future is more difficult, even, than understanding the past. Nevertheless, I expect that Agent Orange will pass away as a public policy issue, although it will remain very real for veterans and their families who think that they were harmed by it. For many people, what they believe now will probably be what they believe when everything that is being done is done. But a consensus among scientists and, I expect, policy makers who have followed the claims, studies, and arguments will hold that no health effects were proved and that, if there were any real effects, they are so rare that they cannot be proved through scientific studies.

CHAPTER 6

AGENT ORANGE AND BIRTH DEFECTS

The warmth, vulnerability, and innocence of a baby make birth defects seem outrageously unfair. A baby does nothing to cause its impairment or deformity. Parents, racking their memories for what they might have done to have caused the disaster, react with self-blame and anger. Even the casual passerby is shaken by seeing an impaired child. Because no matter how much love is shared between parent and child, the passerby cannot look completely beyond the parents' emotional burden and the child's striving against frustration and pain. The parents, moreover, must sustain substantial monetary outlays, great enough to break many unassisted families, for medical care, schooling, special clothes and appliances.

With overtones of disaster striking the innocents, the question of birth defects and reproductive health effects has understandably taken center stage in the controversy regarding dioxin and Agent Orange. The discovery that dioxin causes birth defects in mice[1] propelled the chemical into newspaper headlines. A study associating an increase of spontaneous abortions with the dioxin-containing herbicide 2,4,5-T was instrumental in banning most uses of the chemical.[2] Furthermore, a Vietnamese physician reported that pregnant women who had been sprayed with Agent Orange delivered children with birth defects.[3] More significant to the claims of American veterans that Agent Orange caused birth defects in their children, the same physician reported that children fathered by North Vietnamese sol-

105

diers who fought in South Vietnam were much more likely to be born with anencephaly (absence of all or part of the brain).[4]

Despite the political and legal importance of the several claimed relationships between Agent Orange (and dioxin) and birth defects and abortions, the only one that has withstood scientific scrutiny is that dioxin causes birth defects and fetal death in animals. Even that conclusion has to be circumscribed: Dioxin causes birth defects in mice, for certain, and perhaps in rats, and fetal death in rats, monkeys, and other animals.[5] Furthermore, both effects—birth defects and spontaneous abortions—are evident only when pregnant animals are exposed to dioxin. The amount of dioxin necessary to cause those effects is high, often causing overt health effects in the exposed female animals as well. In any case, these studies have little relationship to the question of Agent Orange and birth defects in children. Fathers, not mothers, were exposed to Agent Orange.

A single study has examined the reproductive effects of feeding Agent Orange to male mice. The mice were exposed to sufficient amounts of dioxin to cause liver and thymus toxicity, and no doubt it made them sick. Even those amounts of Agent Orange, however, had no effect on sperm concentration, motility, or appearance even after eight weeks of exposure. To test the possibility that exposure of males could cause birth defects or spontaneous abortions, the male mice were mated repeatedly with unexposed females. Again, there were no effects: Exposed males mated as frequently as unexposed males and fathered the same number of pups, and there was no increase in birth defects or early deaths among mice fathered by Agent-Orange-exposed males.[6] A 1984 review of the literature on dioxin and birth defects concluded that there was no evidence to prove and little to suggest that exposure to Agent Orange in Vietnam could cause birth defects.[7] Furthermore, a conference of scientists from around the world who met in Vietnam reached the same conclusion.[8]

Certainly results from animal studies and small-scale studies in humans do not necessarily prove that Agent Orange cannot have an effect on the children of exposed men. Primarily, it is impossible to prove a negative—to say that something does not or cannot happen—because at any minute, that something might occur. Looking for that something over and over and not finding it nevertheless makes us more certain that it will not happen, though that is not the same as proving that it will not.

Arguments about the importance and relevance of animal studies come up repeatedly in debates about the effects of chemicals in the environment. So it is with Agent Orange and birth defects. People who believe that Agent Orange causes birth defects are likely to refer to the results that show it caused birth defects in mice and make little of the fact that these effects occurred only when pregnant females were exposed. People on the other side are likely to point to the absence of any reproductive health problems when male mice were exposed and that birth defects have been seen only in mice; not in hamsters, monkeys, or other animals. No matter what data from animal tests are brought forward, they can hardly settle the question; there are limits on the applicability of animal results to predictions of human risk.

How can anyone take seriously claims of no effects based on studies of mice, when there exist stories of devastating effects in humans? For instance, Michael Uhl and Tod Ensign, in a book about veterans exposed to Agent Orange,[9] report the story of a board member of the Nassau County (Long Island, New York) chapter of the Spina Bifida Association of America. According to her, at a 1979 meeting of about 50 mothers of spina bifida babies, the question was asked, "How many of you are married to Vietnam veterans?," to which 35 of the women raised their hands. That would be an extraordinary finding. Spinia bifida, an incomplete closure of the spinal column, is the second most common major birth defect, but it occurs only about once in every 1200 births in New York State.[10] It would be truly extraordinary to find that 70% of such births occurred to wives of Vietnam veterans. Unfortunately, the woman who told the story to Uhl and Ensign would not reveal the names of any of the women who had attended the meeting. She said that the fathers of the children already felt enough guilt and that the wives did not want to get into public discussions of their personal tragedies. Uhl and Ensign commented that they could understand the women's attitude, but that, regrettably, without more information they could not follow up on the story. As far I know, the story has dropped from sight, which is surprising because the meeting took place on Long Island, which was the center of the veterans' law suit brought against manufacturers of Agent Orange. I would have expected veterans who live there to have contacted the lawyers in the suit. Yet, to my knowledge, that did not happen.

In 1979 and 1980, veterans brought forth many cases of birth defects among their children. No amount of evidence from animal studies could convince veterans and many others that exposure to Agent Orange was not related to the birth defects. For a change, the Federal government was able to carry out a study to investigate veterans' concerns, and it did.

The study was made possible through the Metropolitian Atlanta Congenital Birth Defects Program, which registers all babies born with birth defects in the five counties of the greater Atlanta, Georgia, area. The program has the distinction of being the only such registry in the country. The Centers for Disease Control (CDC), which operates the "Atlanta registry," designed the birth defects study and obtained funding for it from the Veterans Administration, the Department of Defense, and the Department of Health and Human Services. The planning and the funding agreement were completed quickly, I think, because scientists and policy makers in the Federal government had wearied of constantly denying or downgrading claims about Agent Orange and, at the same time, being unable to do a study or gather evidence to clarify the issues. The birth defects study was doable in a reasonable length of time, and from the beginning, it promised to provide a lot of information.

The study was straightforward. Between 1968 and 1980, there were 323,421 babies born alive in the Atlanta area; of them, about 13,000 (4%) were born with major birth defects. That percentage of birth defects corresponds reasonably well with the estimate of major birth defects occurring in about 2–3% of babies born alive in the whole country.[11] The variation between 2 and 3% nationwide reflects inaccuracies and inconsistencies in data collection, and the higher percentage in the Atlanta region likely results from the emphasis put on accurate and complete recording there.

The CDC investigators focused their study on 7133 babies with serious defects that are associated with premature death or substantial handicap or that require surgery or extensive medical care. Strenuous and concerted efforts were made to locate the parents of each baby and interview them about a large number of subjects including service in Vietnam. They also interviewed parents of "control" babies—normal babies born at about the same time in the same hospitals. If Vietnam service is associated with birth defects, there should be a larger proportion of Vietnam veteran fathers among the fathers of babies with birth defects than among the fathers of controls. As shown in the table below, the proportion of Vietnam veteran fathers was the same in both populations. While this result cannot prove that there was no association, it clearly provides no support for an association.

The table indicates that Vietnam veterans were equally represented in the groups of fathers of normal babies and babies with birth defects. If that is the case nationwide, we can calculate how many babies with birth defects will be fathered by veterans. Let us accept that 2.8 million men served in Vietnam. If each of them fathers 1 child, there will be 2.8 million children, and assuming that 2–3% will have birth defects, the number of

Vietnam Veterans' Risks of Fathering Babies with Birth Defects[a]

	Total	Born to Vietnam veterans	
		Number	%
Babies with birth defects	4815	428	9
Normal babies[b]	2967	268	9

[a]Source: Adapted from Erickson et al.[10]
[b]Many more normal babies than babies with birth defects were born, but including only about 3000 normal babies in the study was sufficient for statistical purposes.

babies with birth defects would be between 56,000 and 84,000. Frequencies of major birth defects remain essentially constant, so if each Vietnam veteran fathered on average 2 children, the number with birth defects would be 112,000–166,000. These large numbers are a cause for grief; they represent a terrible burden of suffering, anguish, and expense, regardless of the causes, but they show that exposure to Agent Orange is not necessary to cause birth defects. (The high frequency of birth defects was brought vividly home to me when I sat in a hearing room of the House of Representative in November 1984. The Congressman who chaired the hearing, the man who was testifying, the man sitting next to me and I had all fathered children with birth defects.)

In addition to looking at the possible relationship between Vietnam service and total birth defects, the CDC investigated possible associations between Vietnam and 95 specific birth defects such as anencephalus, cleft palate, and clubfoot. None was found. Plaintiffs in the veterans' lawsuit against the manufacturers of Agent Orange charged that veterans' children have been afflicted with combinations of birth defects. To investigate that possibility, the CDC examined the frequencies of combined birth defects, such as all respiratory tract defects and all sex organ defects. No evidence was found to support any association between combinations of birth defects and the child's father serving in Vietnam.

I accept the conclusions from the CDC study concerning Vietnam service and birth defects. There is no apparent association between the two. The results of the CDC study agree with those from an Australian study that found no connection between service in Vietnam and fathering children with birth defects.[12]

But what does the absence of a connection between service in Vietnam and birth defects prove? The charge is that Agent Orange causes birth defects, and not every Vietnam Veteran was exposed. What about birth defects among children fathered by veterans exposed to Agent Orange? Isn't that the important question? Isn't it possible that the absence of an increase in birth defects among all Vietnam veterans' children masks an increase in children of men actually exposed to Agent Orange? The CDC investigated this possibility, but as acknowledged by everybody, it is much harder to determine whether a veteran had been exposed to Agent Orange than whether he went to Vietnam.

Confronted with this difficult problem, the CDC used two different methods to estimate whether a veteran had been exposed. For the first, the CDC simply questioned each veteran about whether he thought he had been exposed. *Veterans who thought that they had been exposed did not father a greater proportion of children with birth defects.* I, and the authors of the CDC study, attach no value to this analysis, agreeing with the generally held conclusion that an individual veteran can seldom know whether he was exposed. He can certainly know that he was in or near a spray from an airplane, but insecticides and herbicides other than Agent Orange were sprayed sporadically. Only rarely would a veteran know the identity of the sprayed material.

The second method that the CDC used to estimate exposure relied on military records. Even so, estimating exposure is such an uncertain process that the CDC still used two variations: In the first, they asked each veteran about which military units he served with and when he served in Vietnam. In the second, they relied on military records for that information. Armed with information about the units in which a veteran had served, the CDC went to an Army records unit, and that organization matched up the location of the units against known uses of Agent Orange. Based on his units' locations and what kind of job the veteran had had in Vietnam, he was placed in one of five "exposure opportunity" categories. The CDC chose its words carefully, skirting the essential question of whether or not the veteran had actually been exposed—that cannot be known (except maybe in a few rare cases).

Since the basic information about which units the veteran had served in was collected in two ways, it is not surprising that the two exposure opportunity indices differed slightly. Although the CDC points to the close agreement between the two indices, the results obtained with them differed. The CDC used a mathematical method called regression analysis to determine whether the frequency of any birth defect increased with more exposure opportunities. If there is any association between Agent Orange and a birth defect *and* if the exposure opportunity indices correctly reflect exposure, then the birth defect should be more common among children fathered by veterans with higher exposure-opportunity scores.

The CDC found that four birth defects were associated with increasing exposure-opportunity scores. Only one, spina bifida, was associated with increasing scores on both indices. Three birth defects—cleft lip with or without cleft palate, coloboma (an incomplete closing of the iris of the eye), and "other neoplasms" (a collection of benign and malignant tumors)—were associated with increasing scores on the index that depended on veterans' recollections. (Also, four birth defects were found to occur *less* frequently in Vietnam veterans' children than in the general population.)

What can we make of these findings? Do they demand that we conclude that Agent Orange is associated with these elevated birth defects? No, not necessarily. Just as finding no effect in a study cannot prove it does not exist, finding one does not necessarily prove that one does. It is possible, and acknowledged by the authors of the CDC paper, that the associations in the CDC study were "false-positives." It is a statistical fact that the chance of a false-positive popping up increases with the number of possible associations that are examined. Since the CDC examined possible associations between 96 birth defects and service in Vietnam as well as possible associations between the birth defects and the two exposure-opportunity indices, there is a very real probability of false-positives in the analysis.

Few people are ever convinced by statistical arguments, but there is also no plausible biological mechanism to explain how dioxin could have caused birth defects.[13] How could exposure of the father in Vietnam cause birth defects? Most birth defects result from events soon after conception, requiring the presence in the mother's uterus of the agent that causes birth defects. While it is possible that dioxin from exposure in Vietnam might have been stored in the father's body and transferred in his semen, that is unlikely, and no experiment has shown any chemical to cause birth defects in that manner. The low exposure of veterans (see the Appendix) makes this mechanism even more implausible. There is an alternative explanation. If dioxin causes mutations, it could have affected DNA in the father's sperm, and that could cause a birth defect. However, there is no convincing evidence for dioxin being a mutagen, although many, many experiments have explored that possibility.[14]

Whether or not the reported associations between opportunities for exposure and birth defects are to be treated seriously depends very much on whether the exposure-opportunity indices reflect actual exposure. The authors of the CDC study acknowledge:

> . . . the estimates of Agent Orange exposure that had to be used were probably rather inaccurate. Therefore, the conclusions regarding possible Agent Orange-associated risks for Vietnam veterans that can be drawn from this study are weak.[15]

Following publication of the CDC results, the Office of Technology Assessment (OTA) was invited to testify about the study before the House Veterans' Affairs Committee. In preparation for that task, my colleague Hellen Gelband and I carefully examined the rationale for assigning veterans to higher or lower exposure-opportunity classifications. As we[16] testified, in our opinion, the CDC birth defects study provides *no* information about Agent Orange. The reason for such a categorical statement is disbelief in the accuracy of either exposure index. Both the CDC and the Agent Orange Working Group (AOWG) have disagreed with our analysis, saying that "it goes too far." They accept that there are problems with the indices, but disagree that they are useless. The most significant measure of the value now accorded the exposure indices is that they are not going to be used in any other study, even though such plans had previously existed.

There are several problems with the indices. First of all, there is not enough information to know that a veteran was with his unit when a spray mission was carried out. Whether he was there or not, he would be counted as exposed. A more systematic bias was introduced by the necessary consideration that a veteran's job in Vietnam might have influenced his exposure. For instance, almost all the men placed in the top two (of five) exposure-opportunity categories were infantrymen. At first glance, perhaps, this appears to make some sense. The infantrymen were moved around constantly, which might have brought them into contact with Agent Orange. But let us assume that two men, an artilleryman and an infantryman, were stationed in a base camp and that Agent Orange was sprayed two kilometers (over a mile) away. The artilleryman would be given a certain score on the index assuming that he had stayed in the camp; the infantryman would be given a higher score. These relative scores would be correct if the infantryman moved from the camp toward or into the sprayed area. But what if he stayed in camp? Or left the camp and moved away from the sprayed area? In either of these cases, assigning a higher score to the infantryman would not reflect actual relative exposures. Finding a weak association between opportunities for exposure that are almost certainly incorrect provides no information about Agent Orange and birth defects.

I have heard no scientist take exception to the conclusion that the risks of a Vietnam veteran fathering a child with a birth defect is no greater than other men's. On the other hand, scientists are split, with a few maintaining that the reported associations between opportunities for exposure and some birth defects indicate an actual connection.[17] These arguments will probably go on for a long time, with scientists trading opinions until they are able to design a study to improve our understanding of the disputed points or the controversy dies. But more important than scientists' reactions to the CDC study is how policy makers have used its results. A representative or senator who considers introducing legislation on the basis of a study must consider the probability that the evidence will convince his or her fellow members who must vote on it. Similarly, judges and lawyers, drawing on their experiences in the courtroom, can decide whether or not the study results are likely to sustain a winning argument in court.

When the CDC results were first made available to Congress, at least one bill was drafted to provide compensation to Vietnam veterans whose children were born with the birth defects that might be associated with increased opportunities for exposure to Agent Orange. However, after careful consideration of the CDC results, the bill was not taken forward. Part of the reason for that decision was the CDC's scientists' careful explanation of their study and its strengths and weaknesses to veterans' groups and Congressional Staff. Chief Judge Jack Weinstein,[18] of the United States District Court of the Eastern District of New York, drew attention to the CDC study and the Australian study mentioned earlier[19] that found no excess birth defects among children fathered by Vietnam veterans. He concluded that evidence does not exist to support claims that Agent Orange caused birth defects.

Some people interpret the CDC study results as suggesting that Agent Orange caused some birth defects. However, policy makers have not accepted that interpretation. Therefore, in the so-far ultimate test of whether the study supports the veterans' claims, it has failed to convince.

We have additional information about birth defects. The Air Force's study of Ranch Hands questioned each Ranch Hand and his spouse as well as an equal number of comparison men and their spouses about their fertility, conceptions, and children. The Ranch Hand study provides information not available in the CDC study. For example, because of the design of the CDC study, no information was collected about infertility, less than desired fertility, spontaneous and induced abortions, stillbirths, minor birth defects, or retarded growth or developmental defects that manifest months or years after birth. The Ranch Hand study examined each of those outcomes as well as major birth defects and found few differences between the Ranch Hands and comparisons.[20]

Of the differences that were found, the two that have received the most attention are excesses of neonatal deaths and birth defects among Ranch Hands' children. Many experts are far from convinced that these differences are real and are waiting for more information. One reason for the wait-and-see attitude is that all the information reported to date depends entirely on parents' recollections. The Air Force is now collecting birth certificates and medical records for all 7399 conceptions reported by Ranch Hands and comparisons to verify parents' recollections. As mentioned before, record verification is standard procedure in epidemiological studies. It does not, in this case, reflect distrust of Ranch Hands or comparisons, but is a check on the foibles of human memory.

But wait a minute. Memories may be tricky, but surely parents would remember neonatal deaths. Shouldn't we regard the reported difference in neonatal deaths as an important finding? Yes; it is an important finding. However, record inspection is necessary to understand the reported finding. "Neonatal death" is defined as a death within 28 days of delivery. Later deaths are classified as "infant deaths." There is a possibility of some misclassification because of parents' not remembering the exact number of days. Furthermore, the difference between Ranch Hands and comparisons appears to be related to a much lower than expected rate of neonatal deaths among the comparisons than to an elevated rate among the Ranch Hands. According to parents' memories, about 1.5% of babies fathered by Ranch Hands and 1.2% of babies fathered by comparisons *before* they served in Vietnam died in the neonatal period. These rates closely parallel the national average of 1.5% for neonatal deaths. About 1.5% of children fathered by Ranch Hands *after* service in Vietnam died in the neonatal period, but only 0.4% of the children fathered by comparisons after Vietnam service died in the neonatal period. The uncertain nature of all information available about a possible relationship between dioxin and neonatal deaths is underlined by the statement of one of the scientists employed by the veterans in the Agent Orange suit: "I'm not convinced without further evidence that there was a causal relationship between Agent Orange and neonatal deaths."[21]

Based on parents' recall, Ranch Hands' children suffered from birth defects more often than comparisons'. When minor birth defects, such as birthmarks, were ignored in the analysis, the difference in rates of birth defects between children of Ranch Hands and comparisons became statistically insignificant. The inspection of medical records is especially important in the area of birth defects; parents may forget to report minor ones or misremember the exact nature of the defects. The Air Force is now collecting those records, but because collecting records for all conceptions in both the Ranch Hand and comparison populations is a time-consuming business, it may be years before we know the results of that analysis.

A third finding has received less attention. The Air Force found an association between children with physical handicaps and estimated exposure to Agent Orange. Just as with birth defects, information from records about physical handicaps may be important to a better understanding of this association, and it is being gathered.

We can expect to see more births to Ranch Hands and comparisons, but nothing like the number already recorded. The men and their wives are aging and passing out of the peak reproductive years; thus, to a major extent, their babies have already been born. Looking ahead, the Air Force examination of birth certificates and medical records will increase or decrease our confidence in the reported associations, but there is little reason to expect any hidden surprises in the nature of big differences between Ranch Hands and comparisons. The information from the Ranch Hand study fits the mold of the conclusion cited by Judge Weinstein that "no laboratory nor epidemiologic evidence exists at this time that is sufficient to link [fetal] deaths or birth defects to parental exposure to herbicides while serving in Vietnam."[22]

The judge left open the possibility that any emerging evidence that either Agent Orange or service in Vietnam caused birth defects can be used in court against the United States. After that decision, some veterans filed suit against the United States as well as against the chemical manufacturers in the Agent Orange case. He dismissed the suit against the government because Federal law forbids veterans from bringing claims against the government. However, he criticized the government as ". . . harsh, unyielding" because it had failed to contribute to the settlement reached between the veterans and manufacturers. He also dismissed suits brought by and on behalf of veterans' children, finding no evidence to support claims that Agent Orange had caused birth defects. Those cases were dismissed without prejudice, however, meaning that the children or their agents can sue the government again if they believe they have evidence of harm from Agent Orange or service in Vietnam.

Several studies have investigated possible relationships between environmental exposures of the general population, both men and women, and birth defects. Federal scientists studied the relationship between the use of the pesticide 2,4,5-T in Arkansas and the occurrence of cleft palates in babies.[23] Their aim was to complement the studies that had shown dioxin to cause cleft palates in mice. They found no evidence for an association. Scientists employed by the State of Michigan investigated claims of increased rates of cleft lip, cleft palate, dislocated hips, and hypospadias (mislocated opening of the urinary tract) in Midland County, Michigan—the home of the Dow Chemical Company. They found a significant increase in cleft lip and cleft palate in 1971–1972, but no other increases that did not appear to be due to chance fluctuations from year to year. Comparable fluctuations were also seen in other Michigan counties that have no chemical plants.[24] In Australia, a special council of experts reviewed evidence that there had been an excess of perinatal deaths among babies with birth defects in areas heavily sprayed with 2,4,5-T. The council concluded that the apparent excess was a statistical artifact.[25] In Hungary, scientists again found no association between 2,4,5-T use and birth defects.[26] Controversy still clouds interpretation of the effects of massive exposure to dioxin in Seveso, Italy, but an international commission of experts has decided that there was no evidence for increases in birth defects there.[27] In contrast, some reports of connections between herbicide use and birth defects continue, for instance, Vietnamese scientists continue to report excesses of birth defects in areas that had been heavily sprayed with Agent Orange.[28]

In the study of birth defects as well as other possible health effects from dioxin, we reach a point where we would all like to say, "Do just one more study. Do it right. And let's clear up the confusion." It won't happen. Humans do not sit still to participate in epidemiological studies, records are probably never adequate to provide certain information about exposure, and even medical records may not be sufficient to allow comparisons to be made between illnesses diagnosed and reported at different times and different places. The perfect study exists only in people's minds. Instead, scientists do the studies that are possible, from which the results have to be sifted and compared. The majority of all the studies argue that dioxin has not caused birth defects. Furthermore, the evidence is more convincing that exposures of American servicemen in Vietnam did not cause birth defects. First, there is no plausible biological mechanism for such effects. Second, exposures were very low, further weakening any biological mechanism that might be invoked. Third, the CDC study and the Ranch Hand study offer no convincing evidence for connections between either Vietnam service or Agent Orange exposure and birth defects.

The absence of evidence pointing to environmental exposures to dioxin having caused defects should be good news. People, including veterans, who worry about having been exposed have no greater risk of having a baby with birth defects than other members of the population.

It is not such good news for veterans who have children with birth defects. They have learned little about causes and are left, as are other parents of children with birth defects, to wonder what might have brought about their personal tragedy. Furthermore, veterans who are convinced that Agent Orange is responsible for their children's impairments can only be further embittered by science failing to support them. Understandably, veterans who have been kicked around by society, "the system," and the VA can see the CDC study and especially the evaluation that it cannot justify compensation or legal claims as another injustice, pure and simple.

One of the possible undesirable outcomes of the birth defects studies is that a veteran convinced that he or his children were harmed by Agent Orange may look on the failure of science to support his conclusion as a choice made by scientists. He may challenge the scientists' integrity and competence. In response to these assaults on their professionalism, scientists can

wall themselves behind their results and conclusions, considering the veterans as data and ignoring them as fellow human
beings.

Veterans who are parents of impaired children are not petty
in drawing attention to their plight or in asking for investigations about possible causes. Now, as the investigations are carried out, however, Agent Orange is disappearing as a reasonable cause for adverse health effects, leaving the origins of the
effects as mysterious as ever. But there is no mystery about the
effects; whatever their causes, they exist. Veterans are ill, and
some of their children bear a continual burden from birth defects. They deserve the nation's compassion and attention, just
as does the plight of other citizens with similar problems.

CHAPTER 7

DIOXIN IN MISSOURI

The United States Government is the largest landowner in the country. National parks, national forests, national seashores, and countless other holdings make up Uncle Sam's real estate portfolio. And while the government has divested itself of some land in recent years, in 1983 it set about acquiring the entire town of Times Beach, Missouri, and some smaller pieces of that state. And it is not because Times Beach is a national historic site, in the traditional sense, or because it will become a national park, or even a retirement community for former Environmental Protection Agency (EPA) officials. Missouri, it turns out, could easily change its nickname from the "Show Me State" to the "Dioxin State," and Times Beach, the streets of which are paved with dioxin, could be the new capital.[1]

Times Beach and more than 30 other sites in Missouri, the others more circumscribed in area, are contaminated with dioxin that all came from the same place: a chemical plant in Verona, a small town on the Spring River in southwestern Missouri. Very roughly, 50 pounds of the estimated 120 pounds of dioxin from the plant's waste have been literally spread around the state. Highly concentrated in chemical sludge, dioxin was taken from the single isolated location in Verona to be distributed around the state and moved from one spot to another, until dioxin could be found in the soil and water of dozens of places. The dioxin levels found in certain places in Missouri were among the highest levels found away from production facilities and waste sites anywhere.

For just over two years during 1970 to 1972, the Northeastern Pharmaceutical and Chemical Company (NEPACCO) produced hexachlorophene at its plant in Verona. Hexachlorophene is a bactericidal chemical that brings to mind the kind of cleanliness that one associates with hospital surgical theaters. Probably most familiar to the laymen as the principal ingredient in the consumer products pHisoHex and pHisoDerm, it was mainly used in treatment of acne and impetigo, cleaning around wounds and burns as a presurgical scrub, and for washing babies. Made from trichlorophenol, it always contains dioxin. NEPACCO abruptly stopped production of hexachlorophene in January 1972, when the Food and Drug Authority banned most of its uses. The ban, ironically, had nothing to do with dioxin.

NEPACCO shared facilities with Hoffman-Taff, a company producing Agent Orange for the Department of Defense. Because both companies used trichlorophenol, the head of NEPACCO, Edwin Michaels, rented a building and equipment from Hoffman-Taff, and Hoffman-Taff employees provided the workforce for NEPACCO. In addition to paying rent and labor costs, NEPACCO gave the larger company shares of its common stock. Thus, a mutually beneficial business arrangement was set in motion. By the time NEPACCO ceased production, Hoffman-Taff had been taken over by Syntex Agribusiness.

NEPACCO made very "clean" hexachlorophene, that is, material with dioxin levels so low that, at the time, they were undetectable in the final product. According to John W. Lee, Vice President of NEPACCO, the company began the process with tricholorphenol that contained 3–5 parts per million (ppm) of dioxin and substantially reduced that concentration to 0.1 ppm. The dioxin removed during hexachlorophene production, which reached as much as one million pounds of hexachlorophene each year, had to go somewhere, and it did. The manufacture of hexachlorophene generates three kinds of dioxin-contaminated waste: dioxin-containing water, "filter clay"—very find clay particles with dioxin stuck to the particles, and "still bottoms"—a thick, smelly residue containing highly concentrated dioxin from distillation apparatus.

The still bottoms, in particular, are a disposal problem. They have to be removed from production equipment and disposed somewhere. When NEPACCO first began operations, it sent the still bottoms to Louisiana for incineration, which was, and still is, the best method of destroying dioxin, but it is also expensive. After that, NEPACCO contracted with the Independent Petrochemical Corporation, a St. Louis firm that supplied them with chemicals, to haul away the still bottom, a cheaper alternative. Independent, in turn, subcontracted the job to Russell M. Bliss, one of the largest haulers of waste oil in Missouri. For the 18,500 gallons Bliss removed in 1971, NEPACCO paid Independent $4625, and Independent paid Bliss $1275. While NEPACCO's officers Michaels and Lee clearly were aware that the still bottoms contained high dioxin concentrations, information about the risk was not passed along the line from them to Bliss. We will never know who knew about the potential danger associated with the still bottom and who did not. As was later discovered, nearly all the dioxin in Missouri's environment came from six truckloads of still bottoms that Russell Bliss's company hauled away. Moreover, the contaminated water and filter clay produced at NEPACCO also mysteriously found their way into the environment.

The contaminated filter clay is perhaps the easiest of the substances to trace, though some may still be unaccounted for. Some was buried at the production site in Verona by NEPACCO, some was taken by the company to a dump that was later transformed into a park, and much of the rest was hauled off by farmers to spread on the ground under the assumption that it would prevent hoof rot in their cattle. On at least one farm, it is know that a flood washed the filter clay into the nearby Spring River; thus, dioxin could have entered the food chain. But this was probably not the first time.

From early on, much of NEPACCO's waste water was fed into Hoffman-Taff's water-treatment system. Inadequate to the task, the system consistently leaked contaminated water into the Spring River. Because the Spring River contamination had been detected by state officials, Syntex, by that time owner of the plant, would no longer accept NEPACCO's waste water.

NEPACCO found an alternative solution in the Water and Wastewater Technical School in Neosho, Missouri, a school that specialized in training people to deal with a variety of wastes. In 1971, NEPACCO paid the school 2½ cents per gallon to accept 225,000 gallons of waste water. Nevertheless, none of the waste water was treated. Instead, most was simply dumped into a concrete-lined basin at a sewage treatment plant that at the time was operated by the school. When the city of Neosho took over operating the plant in 1974, the basin with all its contaminated contents was still there. In 1977, the plant operators began filling in the basin with dirt, gravel, and asphalt, splashing much of the contaminated water up and out of the basin and onto the adjoining land.

The Water and Wastewater Technical School kept about 1000 gallons of the waste water in a tank on campus. As part of their course of study, students would practice opening and closing the heavy valve on the tank. Nearly every time a student opened the valve, contaminated water would pour onto the ground and also onto surrounding students. It was late 1980 when Riley Kinman, chairman of the board of the school and a professor at the University of Cincinnati, personally took a sample of the goo from within the tank. It contained about 2 ppm of dioxin, identical to the average concentration in the Agent Orange sprayed in Vietnam. During the next year, 1981, the EPA moved the tank and contaminated soil from around it to an old Army bunker outside Neosho. The wastewater school closed in 1981, but the building near where the tank had stood is still used today by a community college.

The story of where NEPACCO's dioxin went surfaced in bits and pieces over more than a decade. In all likelihood, most of the dioxin that came from NEPACCO, except the material that was incinerated, contaminated the environment to some degree. But it was the still bottoms that found their way around the state of Missouri to an extent that is almost unbelievable, particularly if one considers that it was at one time all in the same place.

Bliss did almost all his business in waste oil. His company, which he turned over to his son is 1983, purchases used oil from service stations as well as other businesses and resells it to be refined and reused. A much smaller part of the business involves hauling industrial waste, such as in NEPACCO's dioxin-laced still bottoms. Bliss is also a horse breeder; in the 1970s he learned that spraying the floor of horse arenas with waste oil controlled dust. The technique worked so well for him that others hired him to spray their arenas. One application would keep the dust down for months. Since parking lots and unpaved roads also benefited from this technique, Bliss did a fair amount of business keeping down dust.

In May 1971, Bliss's company sprayed an indoor horse arena at the Shenandoah Stables near Moscow Mills, northwest of St. Louis. The "waste oil" sprayed was unusually thick, and left a strong, burning, chemical odor. Beginning immediately after the spraying, and continuing for months afterward, horses, as shown in the photograph below, and a variety of domestic and wild animals became ill and died in the arena's stable. Eventually, according to Judy Piatt, one of the owners of the arena, 62 horses died or became so sick that they had to be destroyed. Even birds began falling from the rafters in such numbers that Frank Hampel, the other owner, spent hours raking them up. Veterinarians called in could not solve the mystery of why the horses and other animals were dying, as though afflicted by a plague.

Hampel, Mrs. Piatt, and Mrs. Piatt's two young daughters, then aged 6 and 10, all became sick with flu-like illnesses during the same period. The younger girl, Andrea, after being away from the arena for a few weeks, returned home and shortly thereafter was hospitalized for severe bladder inflammation and bleeding. All four continued to be sick. Toward the end of August, with the horse problems not showing signs of abating, the upcoming horse shows had to be canceled, beginning the economic ruin of Shenandoah Stables.

During this time, Hampel and Piatt suspected the oil as the source of their troubles. When they confronted Bliss, he assured them that he had sprayed used crankcase oil. Acting on their intuition that the oil was causing problems, Hampel dug up about 6 inches of soil from the entire arena and disposed of it in

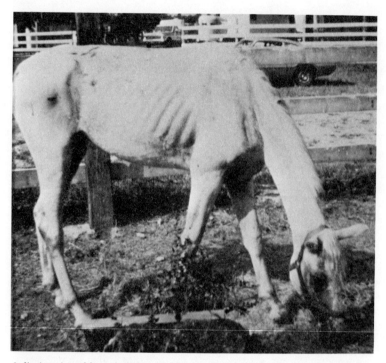

A dioxin-poisoned horse in Missouri. Horses ingested dioxin from the soil when eating and also absorbed it through their feet. Source: Alvin Young.

a landfill. He dug up another foot of soil a few months later. Even after that, when horses were brought in to the arena, they still became ill.

The human illnesses, particularly that of Mrs. Piatt's younger daughter, Andrea, touched off an investigation involving experts from the Centers for Disease Control (CDC) a division of the U.S. Public Health Service. Local physicians had diagnosed Andrea's case as chemical intoxication, but could not find the cause. The first visit from the CDC to the stables was in August 1971, three months after the spraying took place. Though the CDC investigators took blood samples from Hampel, the Piatts, and some of the stricken animals, as well as soil samples from the arena, they were unable to identify the toxicant in the soil or shed any light on the illnesses. Therefore, their report a year later, in August 1972, provided no information about what poisoned the children and animals. Hampel continued to remove soil from the arena in a vain attempt to stem the tide of illness spreading among his horses.

As it turned out, another arena, Timberline Stables, near Jefferson City, Missouri, had been sprayed by Bliss about a month after Shenandoah, in June 1971. Similar problems arose there: 12 horses eventually died, and again, young children became sick. This time, though, the condition of the children was reported to be chloracne,[2] a hallmark of dioxin exposure. A veterinarian who tended the sick animals also contracted a skin condition after handling soil in the arena. However, neither CDC[3] nor Missouri[4] officials have been able to verify that the skin conditions were actually chloracne.

The owner of Timberline, like the owner of Shenandoah, had a layer of soil removed from the arena floor, hoping to remove the problem. Yet the problem persisted. As late as October 1973, the veterinarian at Timberline reported to the CDC that still no progress had been made—and that was nearly two and a half years after the spraying.

But before the next year would pass, the CDC identified first trichlorophenol and then its contaminant, dioxin, from the soil at Shenandoah and Timberline. By the beginning of August 1974, the CDC had notified the Missouri state health department of its findings. By that time, dioxin had already acquired a reputation as the most toxic agent known to man because of its lethality in animal tests. Certain actions had already been taken on dioxin, notably the cessation of Agent Orange spraying in Vietnam in 1971, but dioxin was not yet a household word. Scientists at the CDC, however, among the best informed in the country, knew enough to be alarmed at their finding.

Once the scientists at the CDC discovered dioxin's identity, they wasted no time in trying to find out how it got to the horse arenas, and to find out where else Bliss might have spread his "good will."[1] Two CDC physicians, Dr. Coleman Carter and Dr. Matthew Zack, along with the Missouri veterinarian who had been working on the case since the beginning, tracked the dioxin source to NEPACCO, which by then was out of business. Because dioxin contamination comes from a small number of chemicals, the most common being trichlorophenol, they had concentrated on seeking out sources of trichlorophenol in MIssouri. They found only a handful, and in the end, NEPACCO was the only one that had dealt with Bliss.

A great deal of information about the Bliss company activities had been compiled by Judy Piatt and Frank Hampel, who had surreptitiously followed Bliss's trucks and cataloged pickups and deliveries. Their information proved invaluable during the next phase of the investigation—piecing together the path of much of the rest of the still bottoms hauled away by Bliss.

Of equal importance to finding the whereabouts of the dioxin that spread around Missouri was dealing with the dioxin left in the tank by NEPACCO when it had shut down operations in 1972. That still bottom, containing more than 13 pounds of dioxin in a concentration of more than 300 ppm, was not discovered until 1974 during the CDC investigation. Syntex, the company that took over Hoffman-Taff in 1969, had thought the tank to be empty. By that time, the only accepted method for destroying dioxin was by incineration, but there was no incinerator anywhere that would even be able to handle the 4300 gallons of still bottoms.

Syntex solicited help from the business and academic community, and by 1979, a California company had developed a process to do away with dioxin right on the site. The process was based on the well-known fact that dioxin "photodegrades," that is, breaks down in sunlight because of the action of the ultraviolet light, the same part of sunlight that causes suntan and sunburn. Under the direction of the California company, Syntex built "photolysis" equipment to run continuously for more than three months in 1980. At the end of that time, better than 99% of the dioxin was degraded, leaving less than two ounces of dioxin.

The 1974 investigation continued with Dr. J. Phillips, a veterinarian at the University of Missouri, later to become the Missouri Division of Health veterinarian, leading the charge. Working with the list that Judy Piatt and Frank Hampel had assembled, Phillips found another horse arena that had been sprayed around the same time in 1971, which also experienced similar problems. As at Shenandoah and Timberline, the owners of Bubbling Springs Ranch, southwest of St. Louis, had had the top layer of soil removed from the arena. A road-grading contractor, Vernon Stout, did the removal in March 1973. As Stout explained to Phillips, he had taken the soil to two places: a site he owned on which two trailers stood and to the nearby home of Harold Minker.[1] Soil samples from these sites revealed higher levels than then existed at the horse arenas, since much of the contaminated soil had been removed from the other arenas by then in attempts to end the illness. A sample from the two new sites showed over 850 parts per billion of dioxin—a surprisingly high concentration. It turned out that Vernon Stout had sold some of the Bubbling Springs soil to others along his way, but that was not known until the 1980s.[1]

The CDC, which had done the analysis, and Phillips, working for the state, had warned the inhabitants of the Minker and Stout properties that dioxin was present and that they should therefore minimize contact with the contaminated soil. A more detailed report from the CDC, however, sent to the state and to the EPA, recommended stronger measures: removal of the soil from Minker's and Stout's properties and burial in a secure landfill. But the report also contained a piece of information that was thought to be accurate at the time, that dioxin had a half-life in soil of about one year. That meant that with each passing year, the soil would contain only half as much dioxin, and presumably a safe level would be reached in a few years. So the CDC and the EPA decided to leave the soil in place. Though Phillips took new samples from the Minker and Stout properties about a year later, he did not get the analytical results for another six years, in 1982, apparently because of administrative foulups. The results showed essentially no degradation of dioxin over that year.

By the mid-1970s, the EPA still had not taken a strong role in unraveling the Missouri dioxin story. In fact, it was not until late 1979 that the resources and attention paid to dioxin in Missouri went much beyond the CDC-assisted state effort that has been described to this point. At that time, an anonymous phone caller to the EPA, who claimed to know about the fate of some of the dioxin from NEPACCO, started the ball rolling. The man, who had worked for NEPACCO, met with regional EPA officials and told about the generally sloppy practices of the company, specifically about the burial of drums of still bottoms and filter clay at a farm not far from the plant.[1] Daniel J. Harris led the EPA investigation, following the former NEPACCO employee's lead. A few months later, in April 1980, Harris's team located the buried drums—90 in all. Corroded and leaky, the drums contained dioxin at levels up to *2000 parts per million*. After a full investigation by the EPA of the extent of contamination, Syntex agreed to clean up the site by repacking the drums and sealing the contaminated soil in a concrete-lined area.

Syntex also voluntarily reimbursed the Federal government for $100,000 of the $450,000 that it had spent on investigating the farm site. The Federal government sued NEPACCO and its officers, Edwin Michaels and John W. Lee, for the remainder. The case was heard in 1983, the first such case to be tried in Missouri. The Federal government was awarded its costs.

Following this investigation, the EPA team began probing the whereabouts of dioxin at the Neosho School as well as the filter clay that had been taken off by ranchers to spread on their land. It was only then—not until 1981—that those events were clarified.

In 1981, Harris, leading the EPA investigation, brought back the names Minker and Stout. After examining the farm site as well as the locations near the Verona plant, he suspected that the conventional wisdom regarding the half-life of dioxin in soil was wrong. It had to be much longer than a year. He recommended reconsidering action on the Minker and Stout properties and tried to get help from outside the regional EPA capabilities. Although a Federal EPA Dioxin Task Force had been set up in 1979, Harris's request for assistance from them was essentially turned down. Late in 1981, regional EPA officials tried cutting down the scope of activities in Missouri, but Harris persevered. He was subsequently replaced as head of the investigation. Though no longer its leader, he continued working as part of the team.

In mid-1982, Harris and other EPA investigators visited and took samples from the original sites in eastern Missouri: the horse arenas, the Minker and Stout properties, and other surrounding areas. Analyses found dioxin at concentrations as high as 1.8 ppm in some of the material taken from Shenandoah Stables—more than 10 years after the spraying. The EPA officials asked the owners of the horse arenas to close them and asked the people living on the Minker and Stout sites to avoid contact with the soil. Regional EPA officials shortly thereafter announced an expanded effort in sampling dioxin sites and again tried to draw the Federal EPA more deeply into the investigation.

The Environmental Defense Fund, a public interest group, brought dioxin to the attention of the public in Missouri late in 1982, by publishing a list of 14 confirmed and 41 possible dioxin sites in the state. Once the information was publicized, other individuals came forward with information about further contamination. The EPA asked Bliss for his records of the period of contamination, but he claimed they had been destroyed.[1] Some information from Bliss was on file with the CDC, however, and Judy Piatt's list from her detective days was still available. Mounting public pressure got the sampling program under way relatively quickly this time.

The first site chosen by the EPA for testing was the one encompassing the greatest number of people: Times Beach, Missouri, which is shown in the photograph below. Times Beach was on the list because from 1972 to 1976, Russell Bliss had sprayed the 23 miles of the town's unpaved roads to control dust. Judy Piatt and Frank Hample had recorded these activities in Times Beach, including some dumping of oil, in their account of Bliss's operations.

As sampling got underway pictures of "moon-suited" investigators taking samples from the soil in Times Beach appeared in newspapers across the country. The last soil samples were shipped off to a laboratory on December 3, 1982. It was

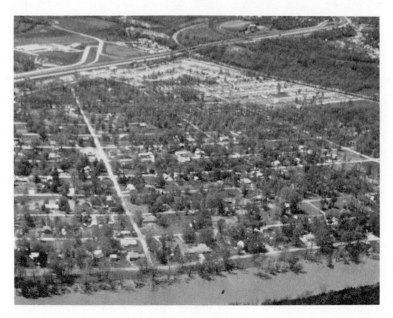

Times Beach, Missouri, with the Meramac River in the foreground. Source: Alvin Young.

fortunate they had been taken when they were, for the following day the town was under water, flooded by the Meramac River. The residents of Times Beach were thus chased from their homes by rising water.

By mid-December, the analyses by the Federal government, as well as some sponsored privately by the citizens of Times Beach, began coming in: Concentrations as high as 300 parts per billion of dioxin were in soil under the roads in Times Beach, and lesser levels were found away from the sprayed roads. On December 23, 1982, the CDC recommended to the state that Times Beach not be reinhabited: Those who had begun to move back should leave, and those still staying elsewhere because of the flood should stay out. The Times Beach residents learned of this latest disaster for their town at their annual Christmas party.[4] Though the recommendation was made public, EPA officials in Washington had not been informed. There was tremendous confusion and uncertainty on the part of all parties. No permanent solutions were set forth yet. Quickly, however, Missouri Senators Danforth and Eagleton, and U.S. and state representatives from Missouri, began to bring pressure on the Federal government to act.

Interest grew within the White House, as pressure from without mounted. President Reagan thus set up a presidential task force on Times Beach as of early January 1983. Members included representatives of the EPA, the Federal Emergency Management Administration (FEMA), the CDC, and the Army Corps of Engineers. The task force was to deal with the dual problems of flooding and dioxin. Lee Thomas, then Deputy Administrator of the FEMA (named head of the EPA in 1984), was appointed chairman of the task force. Rita Lavelle, then in charge of the EPA's activities related to toxic dumps, represented the EPA as one of its two members on the team.

Thomas took charge, making a personal visit to Times Beach to inspect the damage, and thereafter holding daily telephone meetings to coordinate actions of the various agencies working there. Competing political pressures from other sites in Missouri and internal problems within the EPA hampered his efforts. Rita Lavelle held firmly to her position of not taking action in Times Beach until all the evidence was in and of opposing temporary measures, such as temporary relocation. Less than a month after the task force was established, Lavelle was fired by EPA Administrator Anne Gorsuch, who herself would later resign.

Postflood testing results showed continued contamination in Times Beach, but interestingly, the flood waters had not removed dioxin or the dioxin-contaminated soil from the roadways. The presidential task force was thus prepared to agree with the CDC recommendation that Times Beach not be reinhabited because of the high concentrations along the roads and possibly other contaminated areas. Hence, the first Federal buyout of a town loomed. The CDC had previously announced that its leading dioxin scientist, Dr. Renate Kimbrough, had pressed for a clean-up standard of 1 ppb at the Minker and Stout sites; once accomplished, that soil would then be covered with dioxin-free soil. Such a standard would clearly be all but impossible in Times Beach, considering the enormous expanse of road areas that had been sprayed for dust control.

Near the end of February, on the weekend that Anne Gorsuch was married, becoming Anne Burford, the CDC recommended that Times Beach be vacated altogether. By that time, Mrs. Burford and the White House had agreed that a buyout was the only course available to the government. At a news conference on February 22 in St. Louis, Mrs. Burford personally made the announcement that the homes and businesses that constituted Times Beach would be bought out. The Federal government would pick up 90% of the tab—$33 million—and the state would be responsible for the remaining $3.7 million. Although the Federal government initially resisted, similar buyouts were arranged for the residents of the Minker and Stout sites.

Lee Thomas assumed Rita Lavelle's old job, and shortly after Mrs. Burford and many of those working for her resigned from the EPA under the crush of congressional investigations and charges of misconduct. The details of the buyout were left to the remaining EPA and Missouri state officials. Technical problems concerning who would take title to the land and the appraisal of property delayed the process, but offers were finally made to homeowners and businesses beginning in late summer 1983. The government began issuing the first checks about a month later. Plans for all the other Missouri dioxin sites, more than 30 altogether, have proceeded on varying schedules. As of July 1985, the Times Beach buyout was not complete. One elderly couple refused to sell. But more commonly, questions of deeds and titles that can plague the buying of a single house have tied up many transactions, giving realtors and attorneys a lot of business in Times Beach. A problem that will remain after the buyout is complete is what the State of Missouri will do with an abandoned town. One suggestion is to level, pave, and turn it into an airport with terminals and hangers located away from the sites of highest contamination.

As for NEPACCO and Russell Bliss, there was no law controlling the disposal of hazardous waste when NEPACCO produced hexachlorophene and Russell Bliss disposed of the still bottoms, and others disposed of waste water and filter clay. The stringent Federal Resource Conservation and Recovery Act, requiring "cradle to grave" accounting for hazardous chemicals, was not passed until 1976, and it was several years before regulations made the law effective. Missouri passed a similar state law in 1977. Another Federal law, the Comprehensive Environmental Response, Compensation, and Liability Act—otherwise known as "Superfund" because it provides funds for cleaning up toxic waste sites—was passed only in 1980. It provided the money just in time for the citizens of Times Beach to be brought out and to pay for surveys of their health.

There is one thing missing from the story of Times Beach thus far. Such a story does not happen in America without lawsuits. Literally thousands of lawsuits have been filed against NEPACCO and its officers, against Syntex, against Russell Bliss, and all the intermediaries who had anything whatsoever to do with dioxin being spread around Missouri. As sure as dioxin will linger in Times Beach, those lawsuits will be in the courts for years to come. A citizens' class action suit against the Federal government was dismissed by the Seventh Circuit Court, and the dismissal was upheld on appeal.[5] It is likely, though never certain, that the remaining 1400 citizens' suits against the Federal government will either be dismissed or be settled in favor of the government.

Conditions in Missouri, and especially the buyout of Times Beach, focused national attention on dioxin as never before and brought the Federal EPA to the forefront of dioxin control activities. The EPA's actions and plans nationwide in the past few years have been based largely on the lessons learned in Missouri, though there is still work to be done there. In addition, the CDC's safe level of 1 ppb in soil, although developed especially for the conditions of Times Beach, has become the touchstone for all environmental monitoring in the United States.

The CDC is using some of the money provided by the Superfund to establish registries (lists of names and addresses) of dioxin-exposed people. As of the summer of 1985, the CDC had identified between 4000 and 6000 Missouri residents who might have been exposed. Knowing their names and addresses facilitated the CDC's contacting them with information about health risks and to examine them if that is deemed necessary. In a preliminary survey, the CDC examined about 100 Times Beach residents and a comparison group of about 200 unexposed people.[3] The study[6] found no health problems related to dioxin exposure.

Although health effects are limited or perhaps absent, the Times Beach episode had a harmful effect on people. Forced to move, people from Times Beach were seen as somehow contaminated by their new neighbors. In some cases, parents have forbidden their children to play with children who used to live in Times Beach. To paraphrase a Times Beach mother, "Even if it didn't make us sick, dioxin has hurt everyone here."[4]

CHAPTER 8

2,4,5-T: THE UNITED STATES' DISAPPEARING HERBICIDE

In 1948, a few years after its development, the pesticide 2,4,5-T was registered for use as an herbicide by the U.S. Department of Agriculture (USDA) under provisions of the Federal Insecticide, Fungicide, and Rodenticide Act (FIFRA). Farmers immediately recognized its usefulness for killing off broadleaf plants. They relied on it to control undesirable plants in pasturelands, thereby giving desirable grasses a competitive advantage. Rice growers used it to kill weeds in their fields without harming their crop. Foresters also benefited from its many uses: eliminating competing weeds and keeping down brush and shrub undergrowth in coniferous forests. Governments, railroads, and utility companies used it to clear brush from rights-of-way (trails, areas under utility lines, and shoulders of roadways and railroads) without labor-intensive hand clearing. Moreover, it was quick and easy to apply; helicopters and crop duster airplanes could blanket enormous areas with it in a relatively short time. Of course, the Department of Defense gave 2,4,5-T its biggest boost by mixing it with 2,4-D, a related herbicide, to produce Agent Orange, the most famous defoliant of them all.

In addition to being effective, 2,4,5-T had the virtue of being reasonably priced; thus, a large market clamored for it through the early 1970s, making it one of the most widely used herbicides in the United States. In 1974, an estimated 4 million pounds of 2,4,5-T was used for clearing rights-of-way for roads, railroads, and other thoroughfares; 1.5–2.3 million pounds to kill weeds on rangeland; a quarter of a million pounds to control broadleaf pests plants in rice crops; and 50,000 pounds for a variety of uses in forestry.[1]

Over the years, 2,4,5-T was subject to various regulatory actions, some general ones applying to all pesticides that tightened up requirements for safety and rules for application, and some specific to it alone. The biggest concern about 2,4,5-T centered around the dioxin that it always contained. In the 1950s and 1960s, levels of 30–40 parts per million (ppm) of dioxin were not uncommon in 2,4,5-T. Those levels came down after scientists discovered that dioxin caused chloracne in workers and a number of toxic effects in animals. By 1971, many manufacturers had reduced dioxin concentrations to below 1 ppm.

In early 1970, following reports that dioxin caused birth defects and fetal death in laboratory animals, the USDA suspended use of 2,4,5-T in lakes, ponds, on ditch banks, and around homes and recreation areas and canceled all 2,4,5-T uses on human food crops. Two manufacturers, Dow Chemical and Hercules Incorporated, exercised their right under the FIFRA to petition for a review of the cancellation for use on rice. An advisory committee of scientists carried out the review and, in May 1971, recommended that 2,4,5-T use be allowed in forestry, rangeland, rights-of-way, and on rice if dioxin was limited to 0.1 ppm. The committee also recommended reconsidering the situation when there was more information about dioxin's toxicity.

Around the time of the 1970 USDA activity, responsibility for regulating pesticides shifted to the newly formed Environmental Protection Agency (EPA). The EPA took over registration of every pesticide, including herbicides, used in the United States. Under the FIFRA, the EPA is charged with "balancing" a pesticide's potential risks to the environment and humans against its benefits in deciding whether or not to register it (allow its use) for particular uses. If the risks exceed the benefits of particular uses, the EPA can restrict or ban those uses.

In April 1978,[2] the EPA announced that it was considering canceling all uses of 2,4,5-T* and other herbicides that were

---

*2,4,5-T, as used here, also refers to the closely related herbicide Silvex, which also contains dioxin.

manufactured from trichlorophenol. At that time, the EPA's only information about dioxin was from animal studies showing that it caused birth defects and fetal deaths in laboratory animals. One woman changed that entirely, propelling what promised to be desultory hearings into a potboiler that ended in the eventual cancellation of all registrations for 2,4,5-T. It was not a straight path from her observations to cancellation, however.

In 1977, Bonnie Hill,[3] a high school teacher in the town of Alsea, Oregon, took a course at the University of Oregon in which she learned that dioxin caused spontaneous abortions in monkeys. (The term "spontaneous abortion," in contrast to "induced abortion," refers to expulsion of a fetus by a pregnant female without a deliberate attempt to cause abortion. The term "miscarriage" is often used synonymously.) Bonnie Hill also knew that dioxin was present in 2,4,5-T sprayed in the forests around her home. She had had a miscarriage in the spring of 1975, and she recalled that some young women whom she had taught in high school had also miscarried in the spring months, soon after 2,4,5-T had been sprayed.

By early 1978, Bonnie Hill had contacted eight women who had a total of 13 springtime miscarriages during the years 1972 through 1977. Furthermore, from information she obtained from the Forest Service and private timber companies, she mapped spray locations close to the homes of women who had miscarried. Realizing that she, the other seven women, and their families and friends could not collect all the information that might be important, she wrote a letter to 35 government agencies. Because she was "politically naïve," she did not realize that the EPA was the appropriate agency for her to address, but after she recieved nationwide news coverage, the EPA responded to her letter.

It appears that sheer coincidence brought Bonnie Hill's letter to the EPA shortly after the agency announced its intention to cancel uses of 2,4,5-T. It is unlikely that the events that followed would have unfolded so rapidly or that the consequences would have been so great had the herbicide not already fallen under suspicion, and, of course, without her letter, the EPA might have taken much longer to reach a decision.

Two people from the University of Colorado, under contract to the EPA, visited Bonnie Hill in August 1978. Initially, in a study that was dubbed "Alsea I" (purportedly by the Dow Chemical Company), the Colorado researchers accumulated a great deal of information from nine Alsea women with a 19-page questionnaire. The nine women included seven of Bonnie Hill's original eight and two other women that Bonnie Hill had contacted after she wrote her letter. The questionnaire probed into the lives and habits of the women and their families to ascertain more about their health and about the extent of their exposures to herbicides.

When the results of the questionnaire were tabulated, the EPA asked ten experts to examine them and make a judgment about whether they provided evidence for a cause-and-effect relationship between 2,4,5-T and spontaneous abortions. Not surprisingly, the experts unanimously agreed that it would be impossible to make such a judgment on data collected from only nine women, though they did not dismiss the possibility that such a relationship existed. The EPA agreed with the experts, but made the apparently reasonable decision that further investigation was warranted.

By this time, it was December 1978, only a few months before the 1979 spraying season in Oregon was scheduled to get under way. The Colorado researchers designed, carried out, and analyzed the data from a more ambitious study, all by March 1979, which may have set a speed record in epidemiology.[4] Unfortunately, the study, this one dubbed "Alsea II," raised more questions than it answered.

In keeping with accepted epidemiological design principles, the investigators sought to compare the pregnancy experience of the women in and around Alsea with women in another area, one in which there had been no spraying. The simplicity of this concept belies the near impossibility of finding a truly comparable "control" population for the women of Alsea. The investigators chose an area of eastern Oregon that they felt had a similar, largely rural population. For reasons that are unclear, they also chose an "urban" area, Corvallis, Oregon, as a second point of reference, one that they knew to differ significantly from Alsea in terms of both lifestyle and medical services.

Again, in compliance with principles of good epidemiological design, the investigators had to find some measure of the rate of spontaneous abortions that could be compared among the study, urban, and control areas. They came up with what they called a "Hospitalized Spontaneous Abortion Index," or "HSAI." The HSAI was calculated by taking the number of women hospitalized for spontaneous abortions (defined for the study as spontaneous abortions occurring up to the 20th week of gestation) and dividing by the total number of births in the area.

The investigators also compiled data about spraying with 2,4,5-T in the study and control areas. Some spray information for the Alsea area was already available from the Alsea I study, but assembling more complete data was not an easy task because several different forestry companies and the government had sprayed, each keeping separate records. Whatever the difficulties, it is hard to understand how Bonnie Hill, by herself, identified more spraying episodes than did the EPA study team.

Before going on, it is important to understand some things about the type of study the EPA was attempting. First, spontaneous abortions are notoriously difficult to study. There is relatively little information about baseline or "normal" rates. It is widely held by experts that up to 50% of all conceptions end in spontaneous abortion, most of them so early in the pregnancy that the woman herself is unaware of even having been pregnant. The ones that occur that early are never counted. After four or six weeks, spontaneous abortions are more likely to be detected, but even then they may never be confirmed by a doctor. And if a woman goes to her doctor, the doctor may just examine her in the office and send her home. Or the doctor may send her to a hospital.

The women who are hospitalized are the easiest to count; in their cases, there is generally little doubt that they in fact had a spontaneous abortion. Alsea II relied on hospitalized cases. But hospitalized cases may represent only a small percentage even of all medically confirmed cases. Only two of the eight women who signed Bonnie Hill's original letter were hospitalized, but all had medically confirmed spontaneous abortions. The percentage of all spontaneous abortions that are hospitalized is heavily influenced by characteristics of the population, the medical community that serves it, and the medical facilities that are available. Comparisons of hospitalized spontaneous abortion rates among different areas are valid only insofar as these characteristics are the same. If an investigator decides to count not only hospitalized cases, but also other medically confirmed but unhospitalized cases, the number of cases will be increased. At the same time, the possibility of introducing error by not finding all the cases increases dramatically, simply because it is far more difficult to inspect dozens of doctors' records than a few hospitals'. Even more uncertain are the number of spontaneous abortions that are never medically confirmed. These problems in defining spontaneous abortions are compounded by the fact that reproductive problems are highly personal, and many people may be loath to disclose such information.

A second type of difficulty in studying a possible cause-and-effect relationship between an environmental exposure and a health outcome is the impossibility of quantifying exposure. In the case of herbicides, people standing directly underneath a spray helicopter may in fact be less exposed than people half a mile away, whose water supply may have been sprayed, or who eat wild game from sprayed areas. Investigators have to settle for indirect measures, in this case the number of pounds of herbicide sprayed in the areas where people live.

A study based on uncertain exposure and perhaps an unrepresentative accounting of the health outcome is, to say the least, handicapped. Unless the health effects were so great as to be catastrophic, there is little chance that the results of such a study will be accepted by the scientific community. Alsea II was no exception.

What were the Colorado State investigators' conclusions? There were three:

1. The spontaneous abortion index for the Alsea Study area where 2,4,5-T was used was significantly greater than the index for the Urban and Control areas, where there was little or no known use of it.
2. There was a dramatic increase in the spontaneous abortion index for the Study area relative to the Urban and

Control areas in the months of June and July; this increase followed, by approximately two months, a period
in March and April when 2,4,5-T was used to control
vegetation in the forested Study area.
3. Statistical analyses of these data indicated that there was
a significant correlation between the amounts of 2,4,5-T
used in the Study area during the spraying season and
the subsequent increase in the spontaneous abortion index in the study area.

The EPA's reaction was bold and immediate. On February
28, 1979, Douglas Costle, the Administrator of the EPA, issued
an emergency suspension of 2,4,5-T in forestry, rights-of-way
management, and pastureland covering about 75% of the use of
those chemicals, and virtually all uses in Oregon. Costle declared in the Emergency Suspension Notice[5]:

I am ordering emergency suspension of these uses because
I find that they pose an "imminent hazard" to humans and
because I also find that an "emergency" exists because
there is not enough time to complete a suspension hearing
before the next spraying season.

The Administrator's notice presented the results of Alsea II.
No longer did dioxin stand accused only of causing laboratory
animals to deliver small litters or pups with cleft palates. Now
there were real people, Americans, seemingly losing their un-
born children to the herbicide. That conclusion justified the ban.

In Alsea, Bonnie Hill heard the news of the ban, along with
reference to a study, which she assumed to be the nine-person
questionnaire study. She knew, however, that that small study
was inadequate to permit drawing certain conclusions of
causality. Although she was to testify a year later at EPA hearings concerning cancellation of all 2,4,5-T uses, the EPA had
never informed her, or the Oregon State Health Department
official who had helped her, of the existence of a second phase
of the study, Alsea II. Why she was not informed is not clear.

Criticism of Alsea II was as immediate as the EPA's announcement. The study was criticized by many individual scientists, but the most detailed and damaging was prepared by a

group of six scientists—professors of epidemiology, statistics, forestry, agriculture, and environmental health and an employee of the USDA Forest Service—associated with Oregon State University, which Bonnie Hill characterized as a pro-herbicide institution. They tore the EPA's conclusions in Alsea II to shreds. Each of the EPA's conclusions was refuted with a vengeance[6]:

1. The EPA HSAI [Hospitalized Spontaneous Abortion Index] values are not reliable because of incomplete data collection and failure to account for patterns of and differences in medical practice among areas. Conclusions arising from comparisons of data among the three areas are likely to be in error.

2. The seasonal cyclic peaks seen by EPA in the six-year cumulative data are consistent with a model of random variation. The data are highly variable from area to area and from year to year. The "June peak" in the Study area occurred only in one year of the six-year study and should not be presented as a repetitive event.

3. There is no significant correlation between the pattern of 2,4,5-T use and the HSAI in the Study area. EPA's conclusion is faulty because (1) their data on 2,4,5-T spray use is seriously incomplete and in substantial error, and (2) the "June peak" is based on an event which occurred in only 1 of the 6 years.

While the critics did not purport to "prove" that there was no connection between spraying and spontaneous abortions, they said, in effect, that the data from Alsea II were useless in trying to answer the question.

Who is right? The study was flawed. The Oregon State critique was also flawed. During the cancellation hearing in 1980, Bonnie Hill presented convincing evidence that the critics had erred and misclassified some rural areas as urban, partially undermining their own conclusions.

Neither the study nor the critique has been published in the open scientific literature, so they have not been scrutinized by the scientific community at large. No one has tried to replicate the study or design a better one. On balance, the critics are probably more right than are the original investigators. The study does not prove anything about the connection between 2,4,5-T or dioxin and spontaneous abortions, except that such a study may be impossible to do, given small populations and uncertain information about exposures and outcomes. That is not a surprise.

The surprise is that Alsea II, right or wrong, is largely responsible for the cancellation of all uses of 2,4,5-T. In December 1979,[7] the EPA announced its intention to hold a hearing to determine whether or not registrations should be canceled for all the uses that had not already been suspended by the March Emergency Suspension. The notice states that potential risks do not appear to be offset by any economic, social, or environmental benefits.

Testimony in the cancellation hearings began in March 1980. More than 100 witnesses testified, more than 1500 exhibits were entered into the record, and the transcript ran to more than 23,000 pages. Experts testified about the animal tests on dioxin and 2,4,5-T and about what that meant for humans, others testified about epidemiological studies of Swedish lumberjacks, organic farmers who lived near sprayed forests testified about damage to their crops from drift, and Bonnie Hill and several others testified about spontaneous abortions.

In February 1981, nearly a year after the trial began, the Chief Administrative Law Judge stayed the hearing and strongly encouraged the chemical companies and the EPA to come to a joint agreement, without having to resume the hearing. Little progress was made until October 1983, when Dow Chemical, described by the EPA as "the most vigorous proponent of continued registration of 2,4,5-T and Silvex products" withdrew from the proceedings and requested that the EPA cancel all Dow's registrations for 2,4,5-T and Silvex. Shortly after Dow's withdrawal, the EPA commented[8]:

> Dow's actions suggest that the incentives to pursue this litigation may not be as great as they were two and one-half years ago. It is reasonable to surmise that other litigants share Dow's perspective and may no longer be interested in pursuing the hearing.

The EPA's surmise was correct, and over the following year, the other petitioners withdrew, one by one. Union Carbide was the last company to withdraw from the proceedings in late 1984; shortly after that, the EPA cancelled all registrations for 2,4,5-T. Herbicides derived from trichlorophenol could no longer be produced or used in this country.

After that, the EPA never formally evaluated the mountain of evidence presented at the hearings. While there was no disagreement that 2,4,5-T and dioxin are toxic, no one ever settled questions about amounts of human exposure from forest spraying and about human risks from those exposures. Moreover, the EPA never weighed the merits of the Alsea II study and of its criticisms.

In any case, most uses of 2,4,5-T had already been discontinued under the Emergency Suspension Notice of 1979. As substitutes for 2,4,5-T were introduced, it disappeared from the United States market.

Other countries did not follow the United States' lead, however. Expert panels of physicians and scientists in Australia, Canada, England, and New Zealand have met at various times to consider evidence regarding health effects of 2,4,5-T, including the Alsea II study. After deliberation, each panel decided that 2,4,5-T was sufficiently safe to be used in those countries. Each of these panels had scientists from forestry and agriculture, so the benefits of the herbicides were certainly considered. However, I think that the medical scientists on the panels would have carried the day and gotten the panels to recommend restrictions or banning had they been convinced that the herbicide causes health problems. Sweden and some English counties, on the other hand, have, like the United States, banned 2,4,5-T.

All the expert panels have been dealing with a moving target so far as dioxin is concerned. Although 2,4,5-T at one time contained 20, 30, or more ppm dioxin, by 1979 England's Advisory Committee on Pesticides and other Toxic Chemicals specified that no 2,4,5-T with greater than 0.1 ppm dioxin was to be used, and manufacturers could routinely produce the herbicide with less than 0.01 ppm. The committee, in 1979,[9] specifically answered the question: "Can any of the allegations about the risks attendant on the use of 2,4,5-T herbicide be substantiated?" The answer was no: "Such allegations were not sufficiently documented or, where they have been thoroughly investigated cannot be substantiated." Some of the allegations about health problems had been made when 2,4,5-T contained several parts per million of dioxin. The absence of documented effects at the times of use of "dirtier" 2,4,5-T reinforced the conclusion that the 2,4,5-T with 0.1 or less ppm dioxin could safely be used.

Because 2,4,5-T continues to be used in other countries and because dioxin continues to be worrisome, concerned citizens in other countries continue to ask regulatory agencies for investigations, restrictions, and bans on its use. In September 1983, a justice of the Supreme Court of Nova Scotia decided that a group of landowners had failed to show that spraying Esteron 3-3E, a mixture similar to Agent Orange, would be a hazard to their health. He therefore permitted spraying of nearby forests to continue.[10]

Both the plaintiff landowners and other residents and the defendant forestry company called many of the world's experts to testify on the use, economics, and health effects of 2,4-D and 2,4,5-T. The uses of Esteron 3-3E in Nova Scotia parallel the former uses of 2,4,5-T around Alsea. However, according to the trial description provided by the Nova Scotia judge in his decision, few witnesses spent much time discussing Alsea. Although the reported excess of spontaneous abortions at Alsea was brought up from time to time, the weight of expert opinion that the study's design and data could not support its conclusions told against it, and it appeared to be of little importance. Instead, trial testimony placed great emphasis on the possible relationship between dioxin and cancer.

There were arguments on both sides, of course, but the judge's decision devoted some attention to risk assessment information that compared the cancer risk from being in a sprayed area to other cancer risks as shown in the table below.

The risk from cigarette smoking, which is much greater than risks from the dioxin-contaminated materials, differs from the other risks because it is voluntary. A smoker can choose not

Cancer Risk from Smoking a Cigarette and from Eating Various Foodstuff from sprayed Nova Scotia Forests[a]

Substance	Amount	Increased risk of cancer (expressed as number of extra cases in one million exposed people)
Cigarette	1	1
Berries[b]	1/3 pound	0.007
Water[b]	2 liters	0.003
Deer meat[b]	5 pounds	0.01

[a]Data from K. Crump, quoted in Nunn, 1983,[10] at pp. 119–120.
[b]The risks from berries and water are calculated for materials eaten immediately after spraying; the risk from deer meat is calculated for deer contaminated with the maximum reported dioxin concentration.

to smoke (supposedly, although the problems people have when trying to quit call into question how voluntary smoking really is). A person who lives near a sprayed area is exposed to an involuntary risk; he cannot control his exposure personally. The only things he can do to avoid it are move or convince a regulatory agency or court to stop the exposure. In the United States, regulatory agencies generally do not take action against risks smaller than one in a million. The Nova Scotia judge also decided that the risks below one in a million were acceptable. Indeed, he went further and accepted the conclusions of the defendant's witnesses that neither 2,4-D nor 2,4,5-T nor the dioxin the latter contains at the "concentration to be sprayed on Nova Scotia forests poses any health hazard whatsoever."

While the United States and Sweden have banned 2,4,5-T, other countries have not. The same scientific information is available worldwide and can be considered by each country. However, each country may differ in interpreting the data and in making ultimate decisions about herbicides. The difference in regulatory positions among countries distinctly illustrates that dioxin is partly a technical question and partly a legal and political question.

CHAPTER 9

SEVESO: HIGH-LEVEL ENVIRONMENTAL EXPOSURE

Methyl isocyanate gas from a chemical plant at Bhopal, India, killed about 2500 people in November 1984 and left thousands more to an uncertain fate. Compared to this most tragic chemical plant accident in history, the July 10, 1976, accident at Seveso, Italy, which killed no one, seems, in retrospect, a tame affair. But it did not seem so at the time. About a half pound of dioxin, mixed in a vapor with much greater amounts of trichlorophenol and caustic lime, spewed from the Italian plant and spread across the adjoining area.

Local company (Industrie Chimiche Meda Societa Anonima) officials knew immediately that they had a problem on their hands, but had no good ideas about what the effects of dioxin would be on men, women, children, and elderly people who lived in the area. On the basis of evidence from animal studies,[1] both company officials and local health authorities had to worry about possible outright deaths from exposure to dioxin as well as possible long-term effects—cancer, spontaneous abortions, and birth defects. The events that led up to the industrial accident that released dioxin at Seveso followed the same course seen in other process failures that had exposed workers to dioxin.[2]

As noted earlier, the first step in the production of trichlorophenol involves heating a mixture of chemicals in a sealed reaction vessel, an autoclave. Unfortunate experience has shown that too rapid heating causes a cascade of chemical events that generates unwanted heat and pressure, accelerating the chemical reaction and generating still more heat and pressure. When the pressure exceeds the limits of the seals or safety valves of the reaction vessel, the seals or valves fail, and the chemicals inside spray out. Ironically, the same conditions that cause the excess pressure also promote the production of dioxin, and the explosion-ejected chemicals generally contain higher concentrations of dioxin than are found in trichlorophenol.

When the autoclave seals ruptured in the Seveso plant, the half pound of dioxin descended on an area inhabited by almost 40,000 people. It was a weekend, and as the cloud of trichlorophenol, caustic material, and dioxin drifted south from the plant, many people noticed a nasty chemical smell and closed their windows. Of course, as the mixture of vapors cooled, the chemicals fell to the ground and eventually contaminated about 880 acres. The most serious contamination was concentrated in 215 acres directly south of the plant.

Within a couple of days, rabbits in the area that had been under the cloud began dying and other animals, including birds and house pets, also became sick and died. These animal deaths occurred too soon after exposure to have been caused by dioxin, because even the highest doses of dioxin require two to three weeks to kill. The animals were most probably killed from eating vegetation contaminated with trichlorophenol and caustic chemicals that had been liberated by the explosion, or from grooming themselves after rubbing against contaminated plant life, earth, and buildings. The look of desolation in the area was accentuated because the chemicals killed most of the vegetation that the cloud passed over.

Despite concern about human health effects, nothing much was done to protect the citizens of the area until almost two weeks after the accident. Since many Seveso residents gardened, it is certain that contaminated vegetables were eaten in the few days before the chemicals killed the plants.

There are suggestions that local health officials were temporarily overwhelmed with their responsibilities and that squabbling among local, regional, and Italian government authorities contributed to inactivity, but it is hard for an outsider to know what went on immediately after the accident. In any case, two weeks after the accident, the company that ultimately owned the trichlorophenol plant, the giant Swiss pharmaceutical firm Roche, used a helicopter to map the area and identified the contaminated areas on the basis of plant damage.

The most contaminated area (Zone A), in which 736 people lived, was evacuated, and the people were moved into hotels in late July and early August, about two to three weeks after the accident. Eventually, the houses in the most contaminated part were purchased by Roche and destroyed. A total of 4699 people lived in a less contaminated area (Zone B). There was no general evacuation from this zone, but children, pregnant women, and sick people were encouraged to leave temporarily, and everyone was told not to eat locally grown vegetables and meat. A more distant area (Zone R), in which 31,800 people lived, was not contaminated; it was viewed as a buffer between the contaminated areas and the rest of the world. Also, the inhabitants of Zone R would be an important comparison group when scientists began measuring possible health effects in Zones A and B.

What concentrations of dioxin were spread around Seveso? The average concentration in Zone A vegetation soon after the accident was 500 parts per billion (ppb), or 500 times higher than the level the Centers for Disease Control (CDC) set as a "level of concern" for lifetime exposure at Times Beach, Missouri. The CDC estimated that continuous exposure of a million people for their lifetime—70 years—to 1 ppb of dioxin in soil might cause one excess case of cancer. Since the CDC calculation assumed a direct relationship between dioxin concentration and risk, a concentration of 500 ppb would be associated with an increased risk of cancer of 500 in a million, or an increased risk of 0.05%.

Even though dioxin concentrations dropped as sunlight degraded the dioxin at Seveso, until the people were evacuated, they were exposed to very high dioxin levels. Most important, pregnant women, elderly people, and children lived in that area. Although male workers at trichlorophenol plants may have been exposed to higher levels, only at Seveso were women, old people, and children exposed to such high levels.

No one in the trichlorophenol plant was injured in the accident, and not a single worker developed chloracne. There was no chloracne even in the men who repaired the plant, perhaps because the men, instructed about the hazards of dioxin, wore protective clothing and showered and changed clothes after working in contaminated areas.

These precautions were not taken by Seveso residents who carried on with near-normal activities until evacuated. Within a few weeks, chloracne appeared in people who lived in Zone A, especially among children. Eventually, 183 cases of chloracne were confirmed in Zones A, B, and R, and about 85% of the cases occurred in children.[3] Two factors contributed to the higher recorded incidence in children. First, they are more sensitive, or more exposed through outside play, because several children had the disease even though neither parent was afflicted. Second, health officials made systematic examinations of children, and no such concerted effort was made for adults. About 20% of Zone A children developed chloracne, as compared to about 0.5% in Zones B and R. Except in Zone A, in which 15 of 61 cases of chloracne were classified as severe, all the rest were mild. Although chloracne is supposedly almost never seen outside populations industrially exposed to chlorinated hydrocarbons,[4] physicians reported that in Italy, about 0.5% of children in areas outside these zones and far away from the expanse of the cloud also had mild chloracne. However, common acne may have been misdiagnosed as chloracne in some or all of those cases.

Within five years after the accident, all the chloracne had virtually disappeared, although the 15 people who had had severe cases were scarred. The disappearance of chloracne from the Seveso residents stands in sharp contrast to chloracne that has persisted for more than 30 years in some industrially exposed men.[5] Perhaps the actual levels of exposure were lower in Seveso, or it may be that children recover more quickly. Since 1978, no new cases of chloracne have been reported in any of the zones.

As in all cases of dioxin exposure, chloracne, a recognizable and predictable result, is of less concern than other potential effects. A number of pregnant women were exposed at Seveso, and some were so frightened about the possibility of birth defects that they went to Switzerland to obtain induced abortions. These abortions complicated the already difficult task of trying to determine whether exposure had increased the spontaneous abortion rate. Women who left Italy to obtain abortions—illegal in Italy at that time—may have reported a spontaneous abortion when questioned. In any case, the great problems of measuring spontaneous abortion rates[6] plague researchers whether at Seveso or elsewhere.

The possibility of birth defects frightened many people, not only pregnant women. These fears contributed to the decline in the pregnancy rate in Seveso from 6 to 4.9% between April 1976 and the end of 1981.

Although some birth defects appeared to be elevated (and some declined) in the area south of the trichlorophenol plant, no one knew whether the apparent increase resulted from exposure to dioxin or from better recording of birth defects after the accident.[7] Until the accident, no registry of birth defects existed in the Seveso area; thus, researchers found it impossible to compare the rates seen after the accident to historical rates. That problem is not unique to Italy; in the United States, the Atlanta, Georgia, registry of birth defects, which made possible the study of birth defects in children of Vietnam veterans, is the only one that provides historical rates.[8]

Because dioxin damages the thymus (a small organ near the base of the neck that produces white blood cells important in the immune system) in exposed animals and because the thymus is important in the immune system, a five-year study of the immune status was carried out in children from Seveso, members of the workforce at the trichlorophenol plant, and soldiers who guarded the restricted area in Zone A. Surprisingly, exposure to dioxin was associated with increased immune system activity in children. Although this result would appear to warrant further investigation, none will be made. In the first place, the exposure did not cause an elevated risk by reducing the functioning of the immune system. And in the second, once the study subjects realized that they were not at greater risk, they rebelled against continued participation in studies that included painful skin pricks.[9]

Scientists collected a great deal of data about liver function, neurological problems, and other clinical symptoms in addition to those for immunological effects, spontaneous abortions, and birth defects.[10] Experts were assembled to review all the information. The Technical Committee for the Seveso Accident—a committee of Italian scientists—established by the Ministry of Health in Rome reviewed all the data collected between 1976 and 1981. They concluded: "Except for choracne, no effect on health has been observed."[11]

Since no effects were found in the general population, general health surveillance was discontinued, and studies focused on groups judged to be most at risk. These included people who had active chloracne or history of the disease, the factory workforce, and cleanup workers. In addition, the government established a birth defects registry to collect data from the Seveso area through 1982 and a tumor registry to collect data about cancer incidence through 1995.

In February 1984, the International Steering Committee, which included medical experts from the United States and many other countries, reviewed all the study reports. In summary, the committee said, ". . . nearly eight years after the accident in Seveso it has become obvious that besides chloracne in a very small group of cases, no adverse health effects related to the chemical produced by the accident has been observed." The committee decided that its work was complete except for continued monitoring of the tumor registry through 1995.[12]

The Italian experience at Seveso has been important for other communities faced with dioxin contamination. Italian officials decided to scrape up the highly contaminated soil from Zone A and deposit it in two specially constructed landfills (see the photograph below). The landfills are covered when they are completed so that rain will not cause an "overflowing-bathtub effect," spreading dioxin-contaminated soil around the site. The bottom of the landfill is lined with heavy plastic to prevent leakage, and a drain collects any material that does leak out. The drainage material is constantly monitored for dioxin. The State of Missouri, which has its own problems with dioxin,[13] has gone to the Italians who supervised the cleanup of Seveso for advice

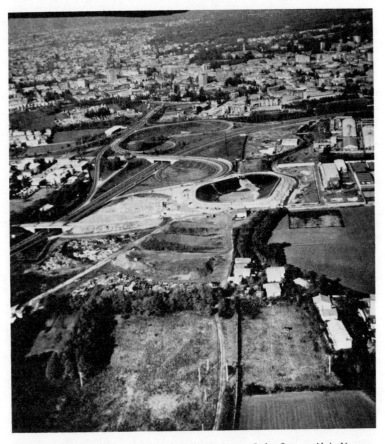

Aerial view of a partially completed landfill near Seveso, Italy. Source: Alvin Young.

about decontamination of buildings and soil as well as disposal of soil that is too contaminated to reclaim.[14]

After removal of the most contaminated soil, clean soil was trucked in, grass and trees were planted, and a park area was established, which has now been handed over to a foundation. Less extreme measures were sufficient to reduce contamination in Zone B. There, repeated plowings of the soil which turned up dioxin so that it was exposed to sunlight and, perhaps, subjected to microbial degradation, reduced the concentrations.[15]

Although pulling up and destruction of plants directly contaminated with dioxin from the chemical cloud at Seveso was an efficient method to reduce the amount of the chemical in the environment, extensive research[16] shows that no or hardly any dioxin is incorporated into crop plants. That good news has to be tempered because dioxin-contaminated dust can settle on the aboveground parts of plants and contaminated dirt can cling to roots and tubers.

The disruption of life around the chemical plant at Seveso was a real tragedy, but health effects have been limited. One death, about two years after the accident, resulted from it. The manager of the chemical plant, taking his child to school, was approached by some men who asked him to identify himself. When he did, they shot him dead. Afterward, a terrorist organization claimed responsibility for the murder and distributed leaflets that said justice had been done for the man responsible for the Seveso disaster.

The Seveso experience, providing a great deal of information about high-level exposure of men, women , and children, suggests that other environmental exposures to lower levels of dioxin probably cause no harm. Conclusions from the experience are already having an impact on decision-making about dioxin. For instance, the judge in Nova Scotia who permitted continued use of 2,4-D and 2,4,5-T in forests[17] referred to Seveso: "Where risk to health might be expected, for example the explosion at Seveso, Italy which caused massive dioxin exposure, none have [sic] been found."

CHAPTER 10

THE NITRO EXPLOSION

A town named "Nitro" seems a likely place for an explosion, but the explosion that put Nitro, West Virginia, on the map was more like a steam kettle blowing its seals than a stick of dynamite going off. Nitro grew up around chemicals. The United States government built a munitions factory there during World War I; later, a rubber products company bought and used the factory buildings. Then the Monsanto Company set up operations there to manufacture a wide range of chemicals, including trichlorophenol and the commercially successful herbicide 2,4,5-T. Until 1953, no one knew that dioxin contaminated trichlorophenol, but dioxin literally burst onto the scene in 1949.

Sitting at his desk at Monsanto on the morning of March 8, 1949, the plant manager was startled by a deafening shriek. Running from his office to Building 41 to find out what was happening, he wondered why no one had activated the steam whistle to alert the factory of trouble. Within five to seven minutes, the noise of high-pressure gases rushing through a vent subsided, and then he heard the whistle that had been on all the time, but drowned out by the sound of chemical vapors spewing up into the air above the plant.

Except for the awful noise, the "explosion" or "accident" or "incident," as the event is variously called, was immediately unremarkable. Safety devices had worked reasonably well, no one was injured, and the accident was not deemed newsworthy beyond the immediate area. But with the passage of time, it became a most remarkable episode in occupational and environ-

mental health, perhaps the most important single event for telling us about the effects of dioxin.

There are at least three stories about the condition of the
inside of Building 41 after the accident. All agree that although
there was an explosion, the autoclave—essentially a 500-gallon
pressure cooker—in which trichlorophenol was being made did
not blow up. Instead, when the pressure inside it built up and
exceeded safe limits, a safety valve gave way, and the autoclave's pressurized contents vented through a stack or chimney
into the air above the building. The plant manager later recalled
seeing a cloud of white vapor drifting from the stack as he stood
outside Building 41.[1]

Accounts differ about conditions inside the building after
the explosion, however. The manager says he saw nothing unusual. According to his recollection, there might have been
some leaks from gaskets on the autoclave, but there were no
splashes of material on the walls.[2] A retired United States Public
Health Service physician, in the course of examining workers at
Monsanto's request—two months after the accident—was
given to understand that the tremendous pressure in the autoclave had bent the vent pipe. Since the bent pipe then ruptured,
much of the contents of the autoclave had spewed into Building
41 instead of outside into the air. According to this account,
when all the material had settled, a white powder covered the
inside of the building as well as the ground outside,[3] contradict-
ing the manager's recollection. Some workers gave a still different account that has received the widest publicity. They contend
that a black powder and a dark brown tarry substance covered
the inside of Building 41.[4] Furthermore, in support of either the
second or third account, a worker four years later reported to an
examining physician that he had helped "clean up the mess,"[5]
which obviously suggests some sort of visible residue within the
plant.

No one has been able to reconcile the various accounts,
although there is always the explanation of the foibles or mal-
leability of human memory. But this is of little importance. What
is important is what happened to the men who worked in Building 41 after the accident.

Within minutes after the safety valve blew, workers were back in the building. The plant manager remembers the atmosphere inside as "prickly," mildly irritating to the skin; he thought that caustic materials from the autoclave were still in the air.[6] In the days to come, workers from throughout the plant were recruited to assist in cleaning and repairing the autoclave and cleaning Building 41. As the workers applied themselves to their tasks, a number of them became ill. Many complained of skin and eye irritations and breathing problems; headaches, dizziness, and nausea soon became widespread. A few weeks later, these immediate reactions to working in Building 41 largely subsided, perhaps because the cleanup efforts gradually removed the chemical cause of distress.

Unfortunately, other, longer-lasting symptoms then began to surface. Three and four weeks after entering Building 41, some workers experienced such excruciating aches and pains in their legs that they were forced to miss work; some even required hospitalization. Other workers found themselves incapacitated by severe muscle pain in their shoulders, necks, and chests, as well as fatigue, nervousness and irritability, insomnia, and sensitivity to cold. A few suffered from decreased sex drive, and some of them became impotent.

Within a week or two after entering the building, workers were plagued with another noticeable symptom; they started breaking out in blackheads and pale yellow cysts. In its mildest form, the skin disease resembled teen-age acne. But on closer examination, it was evident that the blackheads and cysts clustered in a crescent pattern outside and under the eyes and behind the ears—the so-called "eyeglass" or "spectacle" distribution. In more pronounced cases, pustules, pus-containing spots, erupted and spread over other areas of the body, and in some men, the disease caused increased skin pigmentation, giving the skin a gray cast. These characteristics were unmistakable to physicians called in by Monsanto; they knew the workers had chloracne.

Monsanto employed no full-time physician at the Nitro plant; therefore, afflicted workers were sent to various doctors in surrounding towns for treatment. Doctors treated the skin disease with washes and applications of materials to strip away the outer layer of skin; other symptoms tended to diminish as the men were relieved from working in Building 41. However, some of those most seriously ill did not respond to treatment, so Monsanto sent four of them to the College of Medicine at the University of Cincinnati.

Three of these four men had entered Building 41 on the day of the explosion or the next day, and two of them reported that they had been covered with a dark residue inside the building. The fourth man had not entered the building until three months after the accident, but his symptoms were remarkably similar to those of the other three.[7]

Two or possibly three of the four workers had enlarged, sensitive livers and changes in blood levels of certain chemicals that were consistent with liver damage. The liver is, of course, the organ of the body that concentrates a toxin and either degrades it or alters it so that it can be eliminated. However, during these processes, the organ itself can be damaged. Generally, after the toxin is degraded or expelled, the liver recovers to its original state.

The oldest man of the four suffered nerve damage that was visible on microscopic inspection of biopsy tissue. All had chloracne, aches and pains, especially in their legs and feet, and some respiratory distress. The physicians in Cincinnati warned against the men working in hot, dusty environments or around chemicals like those in Building 41. Yet they expected the men, even the one with nerve damage, to improve.

In addition to their common ailments, the men were cursed with a peculiar body odor. When they were in a room together, the physicians noticed a smell that was not the odor of sweat or of the "rancid fat in their skin lesions." The physicians could not identify the smell, but they suggested that the men were eliminating a chemical from their bodies through their skin. If that was the case, and if the chemical originated in Building 41 at the time of the explosion, the men had been carrying the chemical in their bodies for up to six months. There is no way to know what the concentration of the chemical was in the men's bodies, but it must have been high to produce a detectable odor.

Thirteen months after the accident, Monsanto had the University of Cincinnati physicians reexamine the four men. Although the men had improved, none was completely well—some symptoms of poisoning persisted. In general, their skin had improved and their aches and pains diminished. One of the men, the one most nearly recovered, worried about the pain returning, which may be a gauge of how intense the pain could be. Although an earlier report—soon after the explosion in 1949—made little mention of the men's sex lives, a report a year later noted that all had recovered their sex drive and potency. In addition, the later report mentions that the men often felt as though they had gotten sand in their eyes and that two were under the care of physicians because of persistent eye irritation and swollen eyelids. There is no mention of the men's odor in the later report. If the odor had been associated with elimination of a chemical from the men's bodies, evidently the process was complete thirteen months after exposure.

The University of Cincinnati physicians examined two additional men in 1950. One man's chloracne had been treated with X rays. Apparently the combination of chemical exposure and X rays had darkened his skin so much that he was sometimes mistaken for a black man and forced to sit in the back of segregated buses. Being a handsome, proud man with strong racial prejudices, his psychological state declined. His darkened skin caused him to become reclusive, avoiding social and sports events that he had earlier enjoyed. His mental health was so bad that the examining physicians suggested that social and psychological help be provided to him.

All the six men had similarities in their patterns of illnesses, all were improving, and the University of Cincinnati physicians expected their recovery to continue. The physicians' report[8] states that they did not know what caused the assortment of ills.

Despite optimism about the men's improvement in 1949 and 1950, even four years after the accident not all had fully recovered. Of 117 men who developed chloracne after working in Building 41 following the accident, 27 were classified as having mild or severe cases four years later.[9] Eleven of the still-afflicted men were examined by University of Cincinnati physicians at that time. All had improved, including the man with the darkened skin who had been examined in 1950. By then his skin had lightened, and he had married and resumed a normal life. There were no signs of liver damage in any of the men, consistent with recovery of that organ from chemical poisoning. The man with neurological damage was judged to have improved and was reportedly in good spirits, but the physicians were puzzled by his continued lack of feeling in his legs and feet. Two of the four men originally examined in 1949 had not returned to full-time work because of aches and pains. Clearly, some symptoms that were seen soon after exposure persisted for years in some men.

This medical examination, four years after the explosion, reported that 97 other Nitro workers had developed chloracne. None of these workers had been present at the 1949 accident or helped in its cleanup, but many had been involved in manufacture of trichlorohenol or 2,4,5-T. Their cloracne resulted from leaks in the normal process of producing trichlorophenol rather than from a spectacular exposure such as the 1949 accident. Physicians examining 25 of 97 men found that the 25 had symptoms similar to but less severe than those seen in the workers exposed in the 1949 accident. In addition to chloracne, they too suffered from fatigue, aches and pains, eye irritations, and decreased sex drive. The doctors concluded that exposures in routine operations had been to lower levels of whatever it was that was causing the panoply of illnesses.

The numerous outbreaks of chloracne and other illnesses did not go unrecognized by the Nitro workers. Knowing that something in the trichlorophenol and 2,4,5-T processes was responsible, the union negotiated a small hourly surcharge to the wages of men who manufactured those chemicals. Furthermore, the contract allowed men to refuse work in either process without disciplinary action being taken, a unique agreement in the plant.[10]

The 1949 accident, the various persistent symptoms in exposed workers, the continual appearance of new cases of chloracne, and the hazard pay agreement between the union and Monsanto took place before anyone knew that dioxin was causing the problems. As mentioned earlier, dioxin was not identified as the culprit until Dr. Karl Schulz in 1957 identified it as the chloracne-causing chemical in trichlorophenol. Naturally, the demonstration that dioxin caused birth defects and cancer in laboratory animals in the 1970s raised the level of concern about the health of the Nitro workers.

Studies of the Nitro population are now a major source of information about the effects of high-level dioxin exposure. Of all the diseases that have been associated with dioxin, cancer is the most feared, but other diseases, such as heart disease, the number one killer in the United States, are sometimes suggested as linked to it.

Dr. R. Suskind of the University of Cincinnati, who had examined and treated the Nitro workers after the explosion, continued examining the population of exposed men. Making the reasonable assumption that any life-shortening effects of dioxin would most likely be seen in men stricken with chloracne, he identified a total of 121 men who had been present at the time of the explosion and who had developed the disease. It is a comment on the employment practices of the time that all were white. Each man was traced through various records, and Dr. Suskind and his colleague Judith Zack determined that 32 of the 121 had died through the end of 1978, 29 years after the accident. Obtaining a death certificate for each deceased man, they were able to compare the number of deaths in the chloracne-stricken workers with the number expected in the United States male population of the same age.

The total number of deaths, 32, was only 69% of the number expected in a population of white men of the same age. The lower-than-expected death rate reflects the "healthy worker" effect that was also seen in the Ranch Hands: Working populations have fewer sick people and tend to live longer than the general population, which includes people who cannot work because of illness. The death rates from cancer and circulatory diseases, including heart diseases, were 100 and 68% of the expected values. Therefore, 29 years after having been heavily exposed to dioxin, the 121 men had less than the expected number of deaths from all causes, less than the expected number of deaths from circulatory diseases, and the expected number of deaths from cancer.

The conclusions that can be drawn from this study[11] are limited. Because the population of heavily exposed workers is small and because only 32 had died, including 17 from circulatory diseases and 7 from cancer, the study cannot be considered conclusive. Nevertheless, it provides no support for the idea that heavy exposure three decades before had caused excess deaths.

Monsanto Company scientists have completed a second mortality study. Their study differed from Zack and Suskind's in that they relied on company records to identify those who had spent time in dioxin-contaminated areas. A total of 884 white male Nitro workers who had been on the hourly payroll between January 1955 and December 1977 was studied.[12] Females and nonwhite males were excluded because of their small numbers. The dependence on company records limits the study, however. Since no medical records were retained on workers who left the company before 1955, the Monsanto scientists provide no information on any person who had been exposed before, during, or after the 1949 accident but who left the company before 1955. The effect of missing those men on the study is unknown. Nonetheless, Zack and Suskind's study, which traced all men with chloracne from the 1949 accident, assures us that the most exposed men have been studied.

The Monsanto Company scientists obtained death certificates for the 163 of the 884 men who had died. The total of 163 deaths was higher than but not statistically different from the expected number of 158.10* based on national death rates. Deaths from two diseases were more common than expected; bladder cancer was nine times more common than expected and heart disease a third higher.

Exposure to the chemical p-aminobiphenyl, which is not

---

*Epidemiologists habitually calculate expected deaths to two decimal places. If the expected number is less than 1.0, the decimal number provides important information, and I will honor the convention of expressing expected decimal deaths knowing full well that many readers will be aghast at an expected 158.10 deaths.

related to dioxin, almost certainly caused the excess bladder cancer deaths. That chemical, used at Nitro from 1941 through 1952, was shown to cause bladder cancer in dogs in 1952 and was confirmed as a human carcinogen in 1954 by studies in two other Monsanto plants. Many workers were exposed to it during its use at Nitro. A total of 35 men had died from all cancers as compared to 30.92 cancer deaths that were expected. The excess of a little over 4 cancer deaths is not statistically significant; more important, the excess can be explained by 9 deaths from bladder cancer when less than one was expected. There was no statistically significant excess of any other cancer cause of death in the Nitro population.

To estimate the effect of dioxin exposure on mortality, the population was divided between those known to have had opportunities for exposure and those who probably were not exposed. According to the Monsanto scientists, 58 of the dead Nitro workers were likely to have been exposed, 104 were not likely to have been exposed, and the exposure classification of one worker could not be determined. Nine cancer deaths were observed in the exposed group, about two fewer than the 10.94 expected. Although the death rate from heart diseases among all Nitro employees was higher than the national average, and equal to that of the county where Nitro is located, the workers classified as dioxin-exposed had the same lower rate as the national average.

The reason or reasons for the higher heart disease death rates in Kanewha County, where Nitro is located, are not known. An obvious possibility is that the concentration of chemical plants in the county has polluted the area with substances that cause heart disease. Alternatively, or additionally, residents of that county may smoke more or have dietary habits that increase heart disease. Whatever the reasons, on the average, Monsanto workers have the same heart disease death rates as their neighbors, while dioxin-exposed men had lower rates. These findings offer no support for the contention that dioxin increases the risk of heart disease.

The studies of mortality among Nitro workers are important for what they did not find. They did not find an excess of total deaths, cancer, or heart disease deaths related to exposure to dioxin. However, even though the exposed men are not dying at greater than expected rates, questions remain about their health. Did exposure to dioxin damn them to a life of illness and debilitation?

Two groups of investigators reported the results of examining Monsanto Nitro workers in 1984. Dr. Suskind headed one group[13]; Dr. Marion Moses, at the Environmental Sciences Laboratory of the Mount Sinai School of Medicine, City University of New York, directed the other.[14] Dr. Suskind has for a long time examined workers, made diagnoses, and treated workers of the Monsanto Company, and Dr. Moses carried out her study at the request of the union that represents some of Monsanto's Nitro workers. Both Monsanto and the National Institute of Environmental Health Sciences (NIEHS), a component of the National Institutes of Health, supported Dr. Suskind's research, and Dr. Moses's research, which was requested by the United Steelworkers of America, AFL-CIO, was also supported by a grant from the NIEHS. Given the somewhat different origins of the studies, their generally consistent findings are especially noteworthy.

These two studies deserve special attention because they examine the health of a greater number of dioxin-exposed workers than any other study. Furthermore, they report the results of examining men who had been involved in producing trichlorophenol and the pesticide 2,4,5-T since the 1940s. As might be expected from the different origins of the studies, whereas Dr. Suskind depended on company records to identify current and past Nitro workers, Dr. Moses used union records. Almost the entire population studied by Moses were either active or retired hourly wage union members. Most of the men seen by her had worked on the line in chemical manufacture; few were management personnel. Suskind notes that 42.0% of his "not exposed" group attended college, while only 18.2% of his "exposed" group attended college. Despite the difference in educational achievement, the proportion of management personnel was the same in both groups.[15]

In general, better health is associated with higher educa-

tional achievement and higher standards of living. Unless someone can show that the assumption is incorrect, it can be taken
for granted that the unexposed group in the Suskind study
would be healthier than the exposed group on the basis of socioeconomic differences. This situation would be expected to
favor the finding of differences between the health status of the
two groups.

Suskind sent invitations to participate in his study to "all
living employees, active, retired, or terminated." Sixty-one per-
cent of workers classified as exposed agreed to participate in the
study, as opposed to only 46% of the unexposed. No explanation is given for the difference in participation rates, but the
exposed workers were older than the unexposed and hence
were probably more concerned about their health and more
aware of health problems. In addition, the majority of exposed
workers either had chloracne or a history of that disease. With
all the publicity that surrounds that disease, people suffering
from it or who have suffered through it in the past are likely to
be more concerned about their health and more likely to participate in a study. A total of 367 white males—204 exposed and 163
unexposed, according to company records—were examined
and included in Suskind's analysis.

Moses and her colleagues invited 425 workers to participate. Of that number, 226 men completed the examination and
were included in the analysis. Moses and the researchers working with her decided that Nitro workers had moved about so
much in different parts of the plant that available records could
not be used to decide whether a man was exposed or unexposed. Her research team decided to divide the study population between those with chloracne or a history of it and those
who had never had the skin disease. They point out that these
two groups are not exactly the same as "exposed" and "nonexposed," but for their study, the presence or history of chloracne
was taken as a surrogate for exposure.

The percentage of workers who had chloracne or a history
of it was similar in both studies: 49% in the Suskind study and
52% in the Moses study. Men with chloracne were on average
about 56 years of age in both studies. Of those exposed to diox-

in, Suskind found no excess of "nervousness" or "anxiety." This finding is interesting because older people with the skin disease that is known to indicate dioxin exposure might be expected to worry more than others. On the other hand, any worry that was engendered by chloracne when it appeared years earlier might have left the diseased men jaded.

Among men who had ever had cloracne, 59% in Suskind's study and 60% in Moses's study still had signs of the disease at the time of examination in 1979. The disease's remarkable persistence is underscored by the observation that 51 men in the Moses study had had it for at least 26 years, and 29 had it for 30 years! Suskind also found that the skin disease "actinic elastocis" was more common in men who had had chloracne, and it was more severe in those with persistent cases. Actinic elastocis, also called "farmer's skin" or "sailor's skin," is a condition of fair-skinned people that results in swelling of the skin when exposed to sunlight. It is a nuisance rather than life-threatening. Moses found no excess actinic elastocis among the workers she studied. The different findings could result from different diagnostic criteria between the studies or actual differences between the two populations.

Exposed workers more often reported a history of gastrointestinal ulcers than did unexposed workers in Suskind's study of Nitro workers. He also noted poorer pulmonary (lung) function in exposed workers who smoked as compared to unexposed workers who smoked. Although Suskind found *no association* between chloracne (which may be a surer indication of exposure than being classified as exposed on the basis of records) and ulcers or between chloracne and reduced pulmonary function, his findings about these two diseases suggest that the health of these men should continue to be monitored. Moses found no greater frequency of ulcers in workers with chloracne; she reported no findings about pulmonary function.

The most important possible health effects are those that forecast a shortening of life, especially heart disease or cancer, and results bearing on these diseases were generally reassuring. Neither study found an association between either dioxin exposure or chloracne and a history of cancer or heart disease. On the other hand, Suskind more commonly found out-of-the-normal-range cholesterol levels in men with chloracne. This finding is consistent with greater *risk* of heart disease, as are Moses's findings of elevated levels of an enzyme associated with greater risk and higher, although not statistically significant, levels of triglycerides (chemicals of fat metabolism found in the blood) in men with chloracne. For the time being, however, these men show no connection between any of these biochemical abnormalities and increased heart disease rates.

The two studies reported differing results for neurological examinations. Moses reported a significantly decreased sensitivity to pinprick in the afflicted men. In this day of increasingly sophisticated diagnostic procedures, the idea of a physician basing his or her opinion on asking the question "Do you feel this?" as he touches the patient with a pin may seem arcane or at least archaic, but such is the case. However, Moses's analysis did not consider whether or not the men who were less sensitive were smokers or drinkers, either of which can affect sensitivity. She notes that she intends to publish more information on the neurological examination results. Suskind relied on nerve conduction velocity tests, a fancier method, to measure nerve function. In these tests, electrodes are placed over two distant sites on a nerve and an electrical impulse is then generated. The time necessary for the impulse to travel between the two sites on the nerve is measured. Though these tests are also difficult to reproduce, depending on the temperature and humidity of the room and the temperature of the subject, they produce what appear to be satisfyingly precise numerical measurement. Suskind found no statistical differences between dioxin-exposed and nonexposed populations when he corrected for the effects of smoking and drinking.

Both Suskind and Moses found associations between exposure to dioxin and sexual problems in Nitro workers. Exposed men in the former study and men with chloracne in the latter complained of reduced sex drive (libido) more frequently than did the comparison populations. The workers who were most exposed in both studies also complained more frequently of impotence, but the difference was not statistically significant in the Suskind study. Some workers reported reduced sex drive and potency problems soon after the 1949 explosion, and some complaints continued through 1979, when Suskind and Moses made their examinations. The decreases in sexual interest and function apparently did not affect the number of children fathered by the workers. There was no difference between the number of babies fathered by exposed and unexposed men or by men who had had or had not had chloracne. Neither was exposure associated with a higher frequency of birth defects.

As a source of information about the effects of dioxin, the Monsanto Nitro studies have a lot going for them. Some workers were exposed decades ago, allowing ample time for the development of diseases with long latent periods, and many were exposed to significant amounts of dioxin as judged by the appearance of chloracne. There is information about the health of some of the most seriously afflicted men 6 months, 13 months, and 4 years after their exposure, not to mention the two large-scale morbidity studies carried out by two different investigators 30 years after the 1949 accident. The most significant findings show that the exposed men are not dying at rates greater than other men in Nitro and that they do not have increased rates of cancer or heart disease or any other debilitating disease. We cannot be certain that none of the diseases is associated with dioxin exposure, but we can be certain that exposure has not caused any detectable increases in these diseases.

The frequently made statement that the only lasting result of exposure to dioxin is chloracne seems a little glib. The men who were incapacitated by aches and pains after the 1949 accident had a demonstrable reaction to a toxic chemical. Those symptoms, as well as fatigue, eye irritation, and nervousness, persisted for at least four years in some men. Little emphasis has been placed on the psychological effects on those men, but it must have been a terrible source of worry to feel ill and uncomfortable for weeks or months or years and to be troubled with a chronic skin problem that, in some men, meant the daily indignity of having pimples squeezed by the plant nurse. Moreover, serious worry can trigger other health problems. Worrying about health can affect sex drive and potency and reduced sex drive and potency can in turn aggravate worry.

Even now, more than 30 years after the 1949 accident, some of the men exposed to dioxin have biochemical abnormalities that may point to an increased risk of heart disease. We cannot be certain that dioxin is responsible for the abnormalities; it is possible that these men shared other exposures that contributed to the abnormalities, and there remains some uncertainty about whether all the men assigned to the exposed or unexposed groups were correctly assigned. Furthermore, the men with the abnormalities are not diagnosed as ill; some of their biochemical measurements are not exactly "normal," but they are not so different as to indicate disease. Nevertheless, the abnormalities were seen in men classified as exposed in studies designed to investigate the possible effects of dioxin. These findings must be considered when talking about dioxin's effects.

More positive and more reassuring for other people exposed to dioxin and for the many more people concerned about its health effects, there is no measurable excess mortality or overt disease associated with dioxin exposure in the Nitro Monsanto population. That is important because many men were sufficiently exposed to cause serious symptoms shortly after exposure. Although chloracne persisted for years, other symptoms, including aches and pains, disappeared in almost all the men with the passage of time. Studies done in almost two dozen other industrially exposed populations support this generalization, as we shall see.

CHAPTER 11

INDUSTRIAL EXPOSURES
TO DIOXIN

Following the 1949 accident at its trichlorophenol production plant in Nitro, West Virginia, Monsanto made repeated efforts to remove the dioxin that polluted the inside of Building 41. Extensive washings with water and various solvents, burning of surfaces with blowtorches, and painting of all unremovable items failed to eliminate worker contact with the chemical; cases of chloracne continued to crop up. Eventually, Monsanto gave up the battle, dismantled Building 41, and buried the pieces.

The same fate befell other production facilities—in England, Germany, and Holland—where accidents exposed workers to dioxin. Each facility was torn down and the pieces buried or hauled out to sea and sunk. In addition to these three explosions and the ones at Nitro and Seveso, exposures in routine trichlorophenol or 2,4,5-T production have caused chloracne outbreaks in about two dozen production facilities throughout the world[1]; moreover, others may have gone unrecorded.

Scientists have examined the health of the workers exposed in all the accidents and in many of the other exposures and have found results much like those recorded for the Nitro workers. None of these exposures is associated with an excess of early deaths, and there is no consistent finding of any disease or specific cause of death being more common than expected.

Whatever other diseases are linked to dioxin, cancer and heart disease are major worries because they are the major killers. A review of the available data leads to the conclusion that dioxin has not caused these diseases in men present at the explosions or cleanups. No cancer deaths had been reported through 1983 in the 90 men who developed chloracne following an explosion in England.[2] Scientists have examined the number of cancers seen in workers exposed to dioxin in explosions at Nitro,[3] the BASF plant in Germany,[4] and the Phillips-Duphar plant in Holland.[5] No excess of total cancer was found in any plant. The only excess of a particular cancer was three stomach cancers in the BASF population in Germany when less than one was expected. If that excess is actually related to dioxin, there must have been something special about exposure at BASF, because no excess of stomach cancers is seen in other dioxin-exposed workers. Alternatively, the BASF workers might have shared another common exposure that was associated with their cancers, or the cluster of three stomach cancers might have occurred by chance, unrelated to any common exposure.

Scientists found no excesses of heart disease deaths in production workers at any of these plants. However, four of seven heart disease deaths recorded among men at the Philiips-Duphar plant were among men hired especially to clean up the factory after the accident.[6] The cleaners differed from the Phillips-Duphar employees in that they worked in dirtier jobs, going from one factory or waste site to another to clean up situations that regular factory hands were not expected to do. They drank more than Phillips-Duphar workers, for whatever that is worth, and they were exposed to many other chemicals on other jobs. Although the cleaners who died had had chloracne, suggesting dioxin exposure, other exposures could at least partly explain the excess of heart disease deaths. The excess at Phillips-Duphar, not found in other dioxin-exposed workers and limited to cleaners, is more of a puzzle than an indication of an association.

A recent article in the English journal *New Scientist*[6] points out a common problem in industrial epidemiology. The Phillips-Duphar workers are not being followed in any systematic way. Since the company concluded that the men were not at increased risk of disease or death, neither it nor the Dutch government is monitoring their health. Meanwhile, some men who were present at the accident and who are sick are claiming an association. Whether there is an excess of disease cannot be established because all the exposed men have not been examined. It could be assumed that the men who have not come forward to make claims are not sick, but that is a poor substitute for information.

To address the problems of follow-up and to facilitate studies, national and international agencies are establishing registries that include the identities and addresses of dioxin-exposed workers as well as information about their health. The National Institute for Occupational Safety and Health (NIOSH) plans to begin a study of about 450 of the 6000 workers in the United States registry in 1986. The workers' physical and psychological health will be examined, and they and their spouses will be questioned about birth defects in their children as well as spontaneous abortions. In particular, NIOSH will explore possible relationships between dioxin and problems of the immune, nervous, and circulatory systems.

The importance of cancer in considerations of dioxin's effects is neatly demonstrated by the fact that the International Agency for Research on Cancer is establishing an international dioxin registry. The international registry, which is not so far along as the United States one, will apparently include herbicide sprayers as well as industrial workers.

Registries cannot guarantee workers' participation in studies, however. For instance, in 1981, 13 years after the explosion at the Coalite plant in England, the company offered complete medical examinations by noncompany physicians to everyone who had a history of chloracne. Only 29 of 41 men elected to participate.[7] As years pass after exposure, healthy workers may lose interest in participating in the studies. On the other hand, sick workers would probably welcome additional medical consultation, advice, and care if it is available. The result of the different participation rates would be self-selection of sick people into the studies, making interpretation of results impossible.

The one person killed outright in a trichlorophenol reactor explosion died at the Coalite plant in Bolsover, England, on April 24, 1968. The sequence of events leading to the fatality is reasonably well understood. As in all the explosions, a trichlorophenol reaction overheated, the excess pressure burst the reaction kettle seals, and gases blew out. Unique to the Coalite accident, the gases mixed with atmospheric oxygen and formed an explosive mixture that blew up when ignited by an electric light. The second explosion knocked down part of a wall, and the falling masonry killed the chemist.

Dr. George May, a local practitioner hired by Coalite, made two examinations of the company workforce. None of 14 men who had been in the building at the time of the explosion developed chloracne. However, 79 workers who were employed in refurbishing the building eventually developed the skin disease.[8] Dr. May's report, published five years after the explosion, acknowledged the outbreaks of chloracne, but was upbeat in drawing attention to the absence of debilitating diseases that had struck dioxin-exposed workers in other European plants. He also reported that no chloracne had broken out in the plant during the three years following a concerted cleanup operation.

Nine years later, his sanguine expectations for the success of the cleanup had been dashed.[9] More workers had come down with chloracne, and Coalite eventually paid a few hundred pounds to each of the afflicted workers.[10]

The Coalite accident has been well described, but events stemming from it are marked by professional differences, not to mention some mystery. In addition to Dr. May, an immunologist and a biochemist participated in Dr. May's second study; yet they are not mentioned in the report. The immunologist's findings circulated privately, were stamped "Strictly Confidential," and did not surface publicly until June 1983. At that time, Representative Tom Daschle, who has been a champion of Vietnam veterans and their fight for compensation for diseases, released the report at a press conference. The report itself contains no startling information. Although measures of immunoglobulins (proteins in the blood that fight off infections and probably play some role in repressing growth of cancer cells) in some workers were at the low end of the normal range, they do not show that the men are at risk or even that men with chloracne differed from other workers.[11] Had the report been made public when completed, it would have attracted little attention, but its being hidden increased its apparent importance.

Dr. Jennifer Martin, in a privately circulated paper,[12] states that she made the measurements of lipids, enzymes, and triglycerides—some of which, she opines, are consistent with the possibility or presence of heart disease—that are reported in Dr. May's papers. However, Dr. May does not interpret her data as pointing to increased risk. In published papers, Dr. Martin expresses her opinion that measurements made in workers with chloracne have clinical and pathological significance.[13] In my reading of her papers, I found that few of the exposed workers had measurements outside the normal range. Such small pertubations are not generally thought to have clinical significance.

Both Dr. Martin and Dr. Alastair Hay[14] have criticized the conduct of the Coalite company, asserting that the company was slow to publish findings about the workers. Although Dr. May stated that the workers were examined at six-month intervals, he has published only three papers about their health. A total of only three papers is completely understandable if the workers were not sick, as Dr. May contends. Dr. Martin, on the other hand, dismisses Dr. May's interpretations of his results, saying they are intended to be "reassuring," and concludes from her own work that the Coalite dioxin-exposed workers are "at increased risk of coronary heart disease."

In the fall of 1984, I wrote Drs. May and Martin and asked for their latest papers about the Coalite workers. Both responded by sending papers that largely restated their earlier-held positions. Dr. May finds no cause for alarm related to dioxin, and Dr. Martin finds evidence of increased risk of heart disease, but no overt disease. Although it may be too early to draw a firm conclusion about the long-term health effects of dioxin exposure on the Coalite workers, there is not now any excess disease in that population. At least in this country, the Coalite accident is little discussed, reflecting, I think, the general conclusion that none of the measurements made in the Coalite workers reflects any pathology.

Quite apart from differences in interpretation of the biochemical findings, an aura of mystery and conspiracy surrounds events following the Coalite explosion. For instance, Coalite decided that dioxin could not be removed from the heavy equipment in the building, and the machinery was dismantled and deposited at the bottom of an unused 150-foot-deep coal mine. According to Alastair Hay's book *The Chemical Scythe*,[15] the location of the mine has been kept secret even after public inquiry about its location. Although the company has assured local government officials that the equipment posed no hazard, its keeping secret the location of the mine has not inspired confidence.

Also according to Hay, after Dr. Martin had examined all the Coalite workers, the examination records were stolen from her home. Since nothing else was taken, the implication is that someone in the company or elsewhere wanted to prevent her from publishing her results. According to Hay, the police had no clues about the theft.

Coalite weathered the explosion, the questions about the disposal of contaminated machinery, and the cases of chloracne among its work force. Eight years after the explosion, Coalite's refurbished building still stood and continued to turn out trichlorophenol. That changed when the trichlorophenol plant in Seveso, Italy, exploded on July 10, 1976. At the time of the Seveso explosion, Coalite's trichlorophenol plant was closed for its annual down time, but this time it never reopened. Concern that Coalite might blow up like Seveso and spread dioxin across the landscape contributed to the permanent closure of the plant, but most important was the stand taken by Coalite workers. They refused to work in the trichlorophenol facility, and the company closed the building.

Outbreaks of chloracne have not been limited to plants in which explosions occurred. In fact, it is clear that leaks from production equipment or open reaction vessels can expose workers to sufficient dioxin to cause the disease. A cluster of chloracne cases in the United States and another in Czechoslovakia are important because they form the basis for a suggested causal relationship between dioxin and the liver and skin disease porphyria cutanea tarda. This disease is a disturbance in the body's capacity to break down hemoglobin leading to high levels of porphyrins (the part of the hemoglobin molecule that contains iron) in the liver and urine and liver damage from storage of larger than usual amounts of iron in that organ.[16] The urine of diseased people often turns color, becoming pink, dark red, or brown. Sunlight causes the skin of some people with the disease to blister, become "fragile," and easily rub off. Moreover, healing of the resulting sores often leaves scars.

Porphyria cutanea tarda is found in two populations: alcoholics and some chemical workers. The most important remedy is to prevent further contact between the patient and the cause; in the case of alcoholics, they must stop drinking; in the case of workers, they must stay away from the workplace where the chemical is present. Bleeding or chemical treatment to remove iron compounds from the body is the general medical treatment.

The hallmark of dioxin exposure, chloracne, was so common in a Diamond Alkali (now Diamond Shamrock) plant in Newark, New Jersey, that dermatologists visited the plant weekly during the 1960s. A 1964 paper reported widespread chloracne, "fragile skin," excess facial hairiness (hirsutism), and pigment (hyperpigmentation); it also stated that 11 of 29 workers examined had porphyria cutanea tarda.[17]

Seven years later, dermatologists could find no cases of porphyria cutanea tarda among all 73 workers at the Diamond Shamrock plant.[18] Four of the 73 had had porphyria cutanea tarda in 1964, but the disease had cleared up. Whatever had been causing prophyria cutanea tarda had apparently been eliminated from the factory, because there were no new cases.

In a Czechoslovakian trichlorophenol plant, porphyria cutanea tarda has also been reported among dioxin-exposed workers, who bear the unenviable distinction of suffering the most severe and diverse adverse health effects reported for any trichlorophenol and 2,4,5-T workers. Of about 400 workers engaged in the manufacture of these two chemicals at Spolana, 80 became ill during the mid-1960s. Of this number, 55 were hospitalized. Not only did 52 workers have chloracne, but also 38 of them had one or more metabolic abnormalities at the time of their first admission. Hospital records show that the Czech workers had the same problems seen after the Nitro explosion—chloracne, nausea, fatigue, and weakness in the legs.[19]

In addition, 23 of the 55 hospitalized Czech workers had prophyria cutanea tarda. After the workers were removed from the dioxin-contaminated workplace, the disease slowly subsided, and by 1980, abnormalities associated with porphyria cutanea tarda were reported to be "very rare" in the 44 workers still under hospital care.

The findings in the Diamond Shamrock and Czech plants stand in contrast to those in about two dozen other reported dioxin exposures. Excess cases of porphyria cutanea tarda were reported nowhere else. Rather than dioxin, it seems likely that some other exposure(s) found only at Diamond Shamrock and in Czechoslovakia caused the disease. Alternatively, dioxin exposures might have been higher at these two plants than anywhere else, and such exposures might be necessary to cause porphyria cutanea tarda. However, dioxin exposures at Nitro were high enough to cause severe and persistent disease, and no porphyria cutanea tarda was found.

Despite the limited evidence about porphyria cutanea tarda, Congress passed a law that President Reagan signed in October 1984, directing the Veterans Administration (VA) to compensate any Vietnam veteran who developed either that disease or chloracne within one year after leaving Vietnam. Porphyria cutanea tarda provides an excellent example of a common occurrence in discussions of dioxin and health effects. Once an association is claimed to exist, once it is said that dioxin causes a particular disease, that contention can take on a life of its own. Repeated over and over, the supposed link becomes accepted as a truth, persisting in the face of more persuasive evidence to the contrary.

Concern about production workers has extended to their mental health, but the diversity of psychological effects that have been claimed—"apathetic" in the BASF workers and "manic" in the Diamond Shamrock workers—makes it difficult to decide which, if any, of the conditions is related to dioxin. In the Czech episode, the men became so sick that they feared early death; it is reasonable to think that men who were incapacitated by various illnesses would be depressed. As the acute illnesses eased, the men's mental health also improved. The upcoming NIOSH study of American workers is expected to provide more information about mental health.

The idea of "dose-response" is an important factor in epidemiology. Its premise is simple: Higher exposures are expected to produce more pronounced effects than lower exposures. Accepting this notion leads to the expectation that any long-term adverse effects will surely appear in those most highly exposed; in this case, that would refer to industrially exposed populations. As an example of how dose and response are related, let us consider asbestos. All of us are exposed to low levels of asbestos, from flaking insulation in buildings and abraded automobile brake linings, but these exposures do not cause mesothelioma, a tumor on the lining of the chest cavity. This tumor, which occurrs almost exclusively in highly exposed asbestos workers, is essentially unknown in other people. Dose–response relationships are also important in interpreting laboratory experiments. Tests of a substance for carcinogenicity, for example, are more convincing if there is a dose–response relationship, with the incidence of cancer increasing at higher doses. If, on the other hand, the number of cancers varies sporadically with dose, the evidence for the substance being a carcinogen diminishes or vanishes.

We have some evidence to show that dioxin toxicity, poisoning from dioxin, depends on dose, and equally important, none to suggest that toxicity is independent of dose. Although dioxin is terribly lethal in laboratory animals, there are doses that do not kill animals, do not cause cancer in animals, and do not disrupt animals' biochemistry. While several hundred trichlorophenol and 2,4,5-T production workers have been made acutely ill and suffered from chloracne as a result of dioxin exposure, other workers in the same plants have not developed chloracne. The level of the chloracne-free workers' exposure had to be less than that of ill workers, but it must also have been greater than the exposures of people who work farther away from dioxin. Therefore, in humans as well, there are levels of dioxin that do not cause disease. Complementing these observations of workers, a small number of experiments on humans show that very small doses of dioxin applied directly to the skin do not cause chloracne, whereas higher doses do.

From all these observations, we can expect that the most severe and pronounced effects of dioxin will be seen in people most highly exposed to it. Accepting that dioxin toxicity has the usual sort of relationship with dose, the group of people most likely to suffer its effects are production workers, who are exposed to the highest concentrations.

The clearest finding from the studies of production workers is that men who participated in trichlorophenol and 2,4,5-T manufacture are neither dying like flies nor displaying symptoms that suggest that their lives will be shortened. Although many were clearly exposed to dioxin because they came down with chloracne, life-threatening and life-shortening diseases are no more frequent among them than expected. Sometimes observed differences in biochemical measurements are consistent with an elevated risk of heart disease in the exposed men, but there is no excess of heart disease mortality. Certainly continued monitoring is necessary to see whether the observed differences, which are associated with increased risks, are harbingers of increased heart disease. If unusual numbers or types of diseases should begin to appear among the workers, we can expect the United States and international registries to provide timely information. However, many years have already gone by, and the available information about morbidity and mortality provides conditional assurance that production workers' exposure to dioxin has not shortened their lives.

CHAPTER 12

COMPANY BEHAVIOR IN THE FACE OF DIOXIN EXPOSURES

When the explosion took place in 1949 at the Monsanto factory in Nitro, West Virginia, the company, as noted earlier, had no full-time plant physician, so a part-time company physician and physicians in neighboring towns examined and treated the sick workers. But none of the doctors had had specialized training in occupational medicine. At that time, the speciality hardly existed in American medicine at all, and whatever there was of it was on a very low rung on of the medical hierarchy ladder.

Monsanto, realizing that some of the men needed expert care beyond the capabilities of the local practitioners and wanting to learn more about what was causing their sicknesses, sent four of the most seriously ill to the Department of Preventive Medicine and Industrial Health at the University of Cincinnati College of Medicine. With the exception of a few academic centers like the one in Cincinnati, occupational medicine expertise in the United States in the late 1940s was largely restricted to the United States Public Health Service and some states' health departments. Although some of the very largest corporations, such as railroads and steel companies, had medical departments, they were more concerned with the prevention and treatment of injuries than with illness.[1]

After production accidents and exposures, most chemical companies, like Monsanto, did little but provide general medical care and try to clean up contaminated workplaces to prevent additional diseases. Except when prodded by specific puzzling

183

problems such as the illnesses in the wake of the 1949 accident, they seldom devoted significant resources to systematic investigation of associations between exposure and disease.

Until the last decade, and perhaps even now, occupational medicine has made more advances in Europe than in the United States. Europeans have shown more of an interest in workers' diseases from a much earlier point in time, and European countries have led the way in regulating exposures to toxic substances in the workplace. Moreover, company doctors play more of a family doctor role in Europe. Given the difference in importance attached to the subject of occupational medicine, it comes as no surprise that although dioxin was identified as a cause of chloracne in Germany in 1957, United States investigations of dioxin did not begin until almost a decade later.

The mighty Dow Chemical Company of Midland, Michigan, began manufacturing trichlorophenol and the herbicide 2,4,5-T in 1950. In 1964, the company scaled up its manufacturing capacity to meet military demands for producing the herbicide 2,4,5-T to be used in Agent Orange. Thus began a long and difficult relationship involving Dow, 2,4,5-T, Agent Orange, and human health.

In addition to the question of effects of Agent Orange on Vietnam veterans, there are questions about the effects of its component chemicals on the workers who produced them. As the production tempo increased, trichlorophenol production workers began streaming into the medical department with the skin disease soon diagnosed as chloracne. On the basis of a review of records, Dow identified 61 workers who had probably been exposed to dioxin in manufacturing trichlorophenol.[2] Dow classified 39 as having had "high potential exposure" and 22 as "low potential exposure." As judged by the occurrence of chloracne, both groups had been significantly exposed: 34 of the 39 high-exposure group and 15 of the 22 low-exposure group developed the skin disease. Dow also identified 204 workers who had worked in the manufacture of 2,4,5-T; according to medical records, none of those men had ever contracted chloracne.[3] Apparently, at Dow, only trichlorophenol workers and not 2,4,5-T workers were exposed to sufficient dioxin to cause chloracne.

When its chloracne problems began, Dow, knowing that dioxin causes chloracne on rabbit ears as well as in humans, painted rabbits' ears with measured amounts of dioxin in an effort to determine the minimum dose necessary to cause chloracne. Every dose caused the disease, with worse reactions from higher doses. The lowest amount tested, 0.5 micrograms,* caused mild chloracne; 1.0–2.0 micrograms, a more severe reaction; 4.0–8.0 micrograms, a still more severe outbreak. Of course, Dow was really interested in knowing what amount of dioxin caused chloracne in humans, and for that, other tests were necessary. The company contracted with a professor of dermatology at the University of Pennsylvania for a study of dioxin in 60 prisoner volunteers.[4]

Because there are ethical and political implications in experiments using prisoners as volunteers—a contradiction in terms—such studies would not be permitted today. But in the mid-1960s, they were commonplace. After obtaining permission from the prison authorities, the dermatologist asked for volunteers from an approved portion of the prison population. Volunteering was induced by small monetary rewards and also by the promise of breaks in prison routine including trips to the hospital for examination and tests along with the opportunity to see people other than guards and fellow prisoners.

The dermatologist applied measured amounts of dioxin to the skin of each volunteer and covered the wet area with a gauze bandage so the material would not be brushed off. Between 0.2 and 8.0 micrograms of dioxin, amounts comparable to those that caused chloracne on rabbit ears, was placed on the forehead and middle of the back of each man. None of the men developed chloracne at the site of application or anywhere else. Two weeks later, the application was repeated. Again, none of the men developed chloracne, showing that the amount of dioxin necessary to cause chloracne on the forehead or back is greater than 16 micrograms. This result is consistent with Dr. Karl Schulz's

---

*A microgram is a truly minuscule amount, a nickle weighs about 5 grams, and a microgram is one one-millionth of a gram. However, there are about 2×10^{15} or 2,000,000,000,000,000 molecules of dioxin in a microgram.

finding that a minimum dose of between 50 and 100 micrograms is necessary to cause chloracne.[5]

The experiment with a maximum exposure of 16 micrograms of dioxin terminated the contract between Dow and the professor. Yet Dow was interested in testing larger amounts, so the company and the professor considered the next step. Before they agreed on it, the professor went ahead and applied 7500 micrograms to the backs of each of ten volunteers.[6] That amount, almost 500 times greater than the amount used in the first series of tests, caused chloracne at the site of application in eight of the ten volunteers. The progress of the chloracne was characteristic, starting as a rash and proceeding to cysts and pimples. After about six months, it disappeared. No liver problems ever developed.

The disappearance of chloracne within six months is something of a surprise, given the disease's persistence for decades in populations of workers. Perhaps exposure to dioxin and only dioxin is not so powerful a stimulant for the disease as is exposure to dioxin and a hodge-podge of other substances that might be present in a chemical plant. Alternatively, perhaps even 7500 micrograms, the maximum amount used on the prisoners, was less than the amounts encountered by workers.

The large dose used in the second experiment was chosen by a simple expedient: The professor took all the dioxin he had available and split it among the 10 prisoners.[6] The dramatic jump to the much greater dose of 7500 micrograms limited the amount of information that could be obtained; all that could be determined from these experiments was that the minimum dose necessary to cause chloracne on men's back is somewhere between 16 and 7500 micrograms—quite a wide range.

Neither the professor nor Dow published the results of this work. However, a Dow scientist, expressing dismay that the professor had gone ahead to test the 7500-microgram dose, made the studies public in testimony before the Environmental Protection Agency (EPA) in 1980.[6] Dow had not agreed to the 7500 microgram exposure and had discontinued support of the professor's work when they learned of it.

Had the prisoners been as sensitive to the effects of dioxin applied to the skin as some laboratory animals are to ingested dioxin, they would have died (see the table below). Since the "average man" weighs 70 kilograms (about 154 pounds), the dose of dioxin given to the prisoners was 7,500 micrograms/70 kilograms, or about 100 micrograms/kilogram. If the human dermal dose could be compared to the lethal doses in animals, it would show that humans are not so sensitive to dioxin as some animals. However, while we know from laboratory studies that some dioxin put on animal skin reaches and damages internal organs, we do not know the efficiency of that penetration in humans, making direct comparisons impossible. (Note the very different lethal doses seen in animals as closely related to guinea pigs and hamsters.)

In 1981, the EPA tried to locate the prison volunteers by running a news story in the *Philadelphia Inquirer*. About 40 men of some unknown large number of former prisoners responded; the EPA then sent an employee to visit each man. It turned out that many skin tests of many different chemicals had been carried out at the prison in the mid-1960s. Only rarely did the

*Lethal Doses of Dioxin in Various Animals
and the Dose Administered to Prisoners[a]*

Test animal	Dose (in micrograms/kilogram body weight) necessary to kill 50% of animals
Guinea pig	1
Male rat	22
Female rat	45
Monkey	>70
Dose administered to prisoners' skin that caused no effect other than chloracne	≈100
Mouse	114
Rabbit	115
Dog	>300
Bullfrog	>1000
Hamster	5000

[a]Adapted from *Chemical and Engineering News*. June 6, 1983. p. 46.

prisoners know what was tested on them; hence, direct questions about what they had been exposed to could not be answered. The details of the dioxin test, where it was applied and how often, were *too* similar to tests of other chemicals to be distinguished from the rest, so the EPA decided that it could not identify the dioxin-exposed prisoners and thus abandoned its efforts to locate them.[7]

Following the 1964 chloracne outbreak in its trichlorophenol production facility, Dow developed a method to detect minute quantities of dioxin. Armed with this method, Dow was also in a position to monitor other companys' products for the contaminant that Dow was convinced presented some hazard to human health at very low levels. Dow invited other producers of the herbicide 2,4,5-T to its Michigan headquarters in March 1965 and educated them on its new detection methods. Moreover, Dow cautioned them that it would monitor their products and would know the dioxin content of each company's 2,4,5-T. The exact purpose of Dow's obtaining that information is not known, but apparently Dow thought its statement would influence the other companies to reduce their products' dioxin content. Had all the companies done that, the industry would have regulated itself and reduced dioxin exposures. However, not every company followed suit. In particular, both Diamond Shamrock (known in 1964 as Diamond Alkali) and Monsanto continued to market 2,4,5-T with high levels of dioxin as compared to Dow's standard. Therefore, Dow failed in its effort to get the industry to police itself.[8]

A month before the meeting, Dow had considered taking its information about dioxin in 2,4,5-T to the Federal government rather than attempting to force industry self-regulation. In February 1965, a Dow internal memo about dioxin, the cause of the chloracne that was plaguing Dow, expressed concern that dioxin present in 2,4,5-T potentially exposed many users of the product to a health hazard. It also stated that Dow's chief toxicologist would soon contact the U.S. Public Health Service and the Department of Agriculture (which regulated pesticides before the formation of the EPA in 1970) to inform them of the presence of dioxin and the hazards it presented. The company anticipated that it might suffer economically from this course, but it was willing, at that time, to accept those consequences.

By March 1965, however, Dow had begun using the process that the German company Boehringer had developed in the 1950s to control dioxin levels in trichlorophenol. Evidently, Dow was confident that the Boehringer process would reduce dioxin to safe concentrations and thereby eliminate the fear of possible health problems from its products.

Holding up its purer product as an example, Dow encouraged and pressured its competitors to develop better processes to lessen concentrations of dioxon. Dow thought, in fact, that it would gain a significant advantage over its competitors while they caught up to Dow's standards. Given its ability to test its competitors' products for dioxin, Dow thought it could always remind them that they were selling hazardous materials or even tell potential customers that Dow's 2,4,5-T was cleaner. Whatever pressure Dow brought to bear, it did not reduce the dioxin content of all the other companies' products to the levels achieved by Dow.

When Dow called the meeting of 2,4,5-T producers in March 1965, it was confident that it could produce the herbicide with dioxin concentrations of less than 1 part per million (ppm). Previously, the concentrations had run about 10 ppm. In comparison, Monsanto, as late as 1965, reportedly produced some batches containing 50 ppm. Yet a cleaner product did not guarantee that workers' exposures were reduced. According to papers filed in the trial between Vietnam veterans and seven chemical companies that manufactured 2,4,5-T, some workers at Dow were exposed to wastes that contained thousands of parts per million. Ironically, the process that reduced its concentration in 2,4,5-T resulted in its high concentration in wastes. As the 2,4,5-T product was cleaned up to higher standards, the dioxin removed from it became concentrated in the wastes. It thus represented a more concentrated hazard to workers who disposed of it.[8]

Information about Dow's and Diamond Shamrock's behavior in 1964 and 1965 became public only in 1983. This information, submitted as part of the Agent Orange trial, was "unsealed" by the judge in the case. The revelations are less than reassuring about the motivations of the people who ran the chemical companies when it came to the health of their workers. As an editorial in *Chemical Week* put it:

> We do not know all of the factors that entered into the decisions made by Dow, Monsanto and Diamond in the late 1960s. But it will be tough to persuade people . . . that those companies had the public interest at heart. And that may make it tougher for the chemical industry today to persuade the public that it can be trusted, for example, to come forward with unfavorable toxicity data on new products. (*Chemical Week*, July 13, 1983, p. 3.)

Although knowledge about dioxin's toxicity emerged slowly, it had been identified as a cause of chloracne and a contaminant of trichlorophenol in 1957. Thereafter, every manufacturer of trichlorophenol and 2,4,5-T should have known about its toxicity and taken steps to protect workers from it. The questions of "When did you know about its toxicity?" and "When did you do something to protect your workers from it?" have taken on crucial significance in lawsuits brought against manufacturers.

One of these lawsuits has been tried, and a decision has been reached. It was brought by employees and former employees of Monsanto's Nitro plant, charging that exposure to six chemicals had damaged the workers' health. The resulting ten-month-long trial was the longest Federal trial ever held in West Virginia. The six-person jury delivered its verdict on April 30, 1985.[9]

The jury decided that Monsanto was not responsible for the illnesses of six retired workers who had been exposed to dioxin, but that it was responsible for a case of bladder cancer in a retired worker who had been exposed to another chemical, *p*-aminobiphenol.[10] The jury's verdict and its statement about dioxin are refreshingly straightforward.

In finding that Monsanto was not responsible for diseases claimed to result from exposure to dioxin, the jury decided that Monsanto had not shown a "willful, wanton, and reckless attitude towards its workers' health and safety." It did find, however, that the company did not "pursue a diligent course of action in trying to determine the full impact of dioxin on the health of its workers." Apparently the jury decided that the company had done what was expected of it; thus, even though it could have done more, it had acted responsibly in light of what was known at the time about dioxin and about protecting workers from it.

After listening to weeks of testimony about dioxin's possible effects on human health, the jury decided: "Based on the testimony of many expert witnesses, it's clear that dioxin, although not directly life threatening, has nevertheless a definite effect on humans, usually involving the skin, nervous system, and general fatigue."[11] The jury decided that in highly exposed workers, dioxin caused chloracne, aches, pains, and fatigue, but that it did not kill or cause chronic diseases. Though some workers were sick from a number of diseases and others had died from them, including cancer and heart disease, the jury decided that there was no convincing evidence that these diseases had been associated with dioxin.

More lawsuits have been brought against Monsanto and other manufacturers, claiming damage from exposure to dioxin. It is impossible to know what the outcome of these cases will be, but with the Nitro case as a precedent, it seems probable that companies that adhered to contemporary standards of worker protection will probably not be held liable. At least from a legal perspective, companies are not likely to be blamed for the workers' illnesses. The Monsanto verdict, of course, went further than that, refuting any apparent tie between life-threatening diseases and dioxin exposure.

After more than 35 years of known exposure to dioxin in workplaces around the world, the facts on dioxin in 1985 were not sufficient to convince the Nitro jury that exposure causes early deaths, cancer, or heart disease.[12] Other trials are still going on, but I expect that the one at Nitro will be a precedent for others.

The Nitro decision and the facts heard in that case do not still the claims that dioxin causes diseases such as cancer and heart attacks. The claims persist, of course, for the simple reason that not everyone comes to the same conclusions as the jury.

Two sources of information are important to sustaining the claims: One is reports of an excess of rare cancers in herbicide sprayers; the other is evidence for dioxin's extreme toxicity in laboratory animals. We will soon explore each of these topics.

CHAPTER 13

DIOXIN AND SPECIFIC CANCERS

Swedish scientists have reported associations between dioxin exposure and several cancers, including malignant lymphomas,[1] nasal cancers,[2] and stomach cancers.[3] However, none of these associations has attracted so much attention as the Swedish reports[4] mentioned earlier that dioxin exposure of forestry workers caused unexpectedly high numbers of a group of relatively rare tumors, soft tissue sarcomas.* Since these reports were published, nearly all investigations of possible associations between dioxin and cancer have emphasized the possible link between the chemical and soft tissue sarcomas. Little is known about these tumors or about their causes, which may in part explain why the press and some scientists have drawn attention to the possible link. Since dioxin remains a mystery in many ways, one may not need a vivid imagination to see why it is often invoked to explain an even more mysterious form of cancer. In any case, the suggested association affords scientists the opportunity to learn more about these tumors as well as dioxin's carcinogenicity.

Soft tissue sarcomas are a diverse group of tumors that can

---

*Sarcomas, which are tumors that can arise in many anatomical sites, are found in body parts derived from the middle layer—the mesoderm—of embryonic tissues. The mesoderm is the progenitor of muscle, connective tissue, the inner layer of the skin, bone, and some other tissues. The other two types of cancers are carcinomas, which arise in epithelial tissues that line various glands, organs, and the skin, and leukemias and lymphomas, which are cancers of circulating cells.

appear in connective tissues, cartilage, or striated muscle in any part of the body; pathologists have identified over 190 well-defined forms under the microscope. Whereas some are malignant, spreading into other tissues and organs, others are benign and do not spread beyond the tissue in which they originate.[5]

Epidemiologists generally use death certificates to obtain information about causes of death, but death certificates provide limited and sometimes misleading information about soft tissue sarcomas. Experts from the National Cancer Institute[6] have found that only about half the soft tissue sarcomas that were found on pathological examination were listed on death certificates *and* that about half the tumors listed as soft tissue sarcomas were actually tumors of some other kind. Furthermore, soft tissue sarcomas that arise in specific organs, such as the stomach or liver, are more likely to be listed as tumors of those particular organs than as soft tissue sarcomas—which contributes further to their being undercounted. All these classification problems complicate the already difficult epidemiological task of studying these tumors that occur with a frequency of about 0.07% in the male population of the United States.

Before the publicity over the Swedish studies, animal tests had suggested associations between dioxin and cancer, but the associations were vague. In particular, dioxin was shown to cause liver cancer in rats. This finding is not altogether surprising, however, since dioxin is a chlorinated hydrocarbon and chlorinated hydrocarbons commonly cause liver tumors in laboratory animals. If the animal results are accepted as providing any kind of a guide to human health effects, they should suggest that epidemiologists look for excess liver cancers among people exposed to dioxin. When scientists did follow this path, however, they found no such link between dioxin and liver cancer in humans.[7]

Nevertheless, scientists do not confine themselves to a direct correlation between sites of tumors in animals and expected sites in humans. Many scientists interpret tumors of the rodent's liver as a generalized signal of carcinogenicity rather than an effect specific to the liver. Other scientists, citing how prone the rodent's liver is to cancer, think that such animal cancers provide little or no information about human risk. The dilemma about the meaning of liver cancers in rodents is by no means unique to dioxin; this quandry plagues interpretation of results from animal tests of a multitude of chemicals.

According to studies of workers exposed to dioxin through manufacturing of 2,4,5-T or trichlorophenol, no association has been shown between dioxin exposure and an excess of soft tissue sarcomas, or of any other cancer,[8] for that matter. However, these studies, which examined the number and causes of death in populations of workers, might be inadequate to provide accurate information about the occurrence of a rare cancer. These studies, as "cohort" studies, could easily overlook the occurrence of a rare cancer. As an example, let us assume that 100 men between the ages of 20 and 50 were exposed to dioxin. Eventually, if their mortality experience is the same as the national average, between 20 and 25 will die from cancer, and most of these deaths will occur when the men are in their late 50s or older. If dioxin increased the number of cancer deaths but did not cause earlier deaths, we would have to wait until the entire population has reached old age to see any effect. If it actually increased the frequency of a relatively rare cancer, the increase might go unrecognized. Suppose that we expected one case of colon cancer among the 100 workers, and two occurred. Even that would not be convincing evidence for an increase. Instead of reaching a conclusion, either positive or negative, from the cohort study, it would be a more reasonable approach to launch a study focusing on colon cancer alone.

Such "case–control" studies are the usual route for pinning down associations between particular exposures and cancers. As noted earlier, scientists identify all the "cases," people who have been struck by a particular disease, and match them with "controls," people as nearly like the cases as possible but who do not have the disease. Cases and controls should ideally be of the same age, sex, race, and socioeconomic standing. Generally, scientists identify cancer cases from registries of cancers in a particular area or from death certificate information. By questioning the cases and the controls about their lifestyles, occupations, and other factors, the scientists attempt to find some factors that are more common in the cases than in the controls. When cases or controls are dead or too ill to participate, next of kin are interviewed. In the Swedish studies, a history of employment in forestry or agriculture was more common among the men with the soft tissue sarcomas than among the controls.

After a number of soft tissue sarcomas had been reported among Swedish forestry workers, scientists initiated a number of case–control studies. Between 1979 and 1981, Swedish investigators published three papers reporting that exposure to 2,4,5-T during herbicide spraying caused a 5- to 7-fold increased risk of soft tissue sarcoma and a 5-fold increase in malignant lymphoma (a tumor of lymph nodes and white blood cells).[9]

Other studies of herbicide applicators in Sweden,[10] Finland,[11] and New Zealand,[12] as well as that of the Ranch Hands,[13] failed to confirm that finding. Moreover, members of the scientific community hurled stinging criticisms at the researchers who had reported the association. The critics pointed out that there had been ample newspaper and TV publicity concerning the possible link between dioxin and soft tissue sarcomas during the time these studies were conducted. That publicity may have unconsciously implanted a reason for people with soft tissue sarcoma to remember that they had been exposed in some way. The Swedish scientists strongly countered that cricitism. In other case–control studies that examined colon and liver cancer occurrence, they also asked questions about herbicide exposures. They found no association between these tumors and herbicides. They were satisfied that cancer patients and next of kin were no more likely than controls to report herbicide exposure unless it actually had occurred. In my mind, the possible influence of publicity on a link between dioxin and cancer remains a somewhat open question. The publicity, at that time, was about a specific link between herbicides and soft tissue sarcoma, and I do not know whether the public would generalize from that information to an overall link between herbicides and cancer. Furthermore, critics have suggested that telephone interviews of the cases at that time focused on the topic of herbicides; this may have caused the cases to recall exposures[14] more often than the controls.

A recognized expert on the pathology of soft tissue sarcomas has charged that the Swedish investigators may have been incorrect in their diagnoses of some tumors.[15] He criticized the Swedish authors for not having published photographs of the tumor cells, a standard practice in many studies. Because of that omission, he and other pathologists have no chance to compare their diagnoses with those of the authors. The Swedish investigators, in their papers, write that the tumors had been reviewed by pathologists, but they do not identify them or give any details on how these experts conducted their reviews.

In the United States, we have had a striking demonstration of the importance of accurate diagnosis. Soon after the publication of the Swedish studies, American chemical manufacturers and the National Institute for Occupational Safety and Health (NIOSH) searched through their records to see if any soft tissue sarcomas had been identified among dioxin-exposed workers. By 1981, seven cases, many more than were expected, had been found.[16] Scientists at the NIOSH, knowing the intricacies and pitfalls of diagnosis and aware that some workers listed as exposed might not have been, reexamined the information. Microscopic slides of tumor tissue from each of the seven were available, and two separate groups of pathologists were commissioned to examine them. Each group, not knowing the findings of the other, diagnosed the same two tumors as not soft tissue sarcomas. This exercise epitomizes the difficulty of accurately diagnosing soft tissue sarcomas. The NIOSH reexamination also determined that three of the seven cases had probably not been exposed to dioxin at all. In total, the reexamination confirmed two cases of soft tissue sarcoma among dioxin-exposed workers, not nearly so alarming a number as the earlier report of seven.

The NIOSH scientists concluded that information is not available for them to decide whether the two cases are in excess of expectation. The primary reason for not knowing is uncertainty about how many workers in the study had been exposed to dioxin. Consequently, researchers did not know what number to divide into two to calculate a rate. Furthermore, they concluded that there is little point in making comparisons with the rate of soft tissue sarcomas in the United States population because of the vagaries of recording of these tumors on death certificates.

Why did the NIOSH reexamine the data about soft tissue sarcomas? Were they under pressure to show that there was no excess risk? No. The NIOSH has a history of identifying occupational health risks and bringing them to the attention of Federal regulatory agencies.[17] However, NIOSH scientists, like all good scientists, pride themselves on careful work, and they thought the reanalysis of the data was necessary because of the difficulties in classifying soft tissue sarcoma and in determining who had been exposed to dioxin.

Arguments between the Swedish scientists and critics probably sway different people to agree with one side or the other. Although one expert[18] on soft tissue sarcomas has called for a panel of pathologists to review any preserved tissues from the Swedish studies as well as tissues from any other study involving soft tissue sarcomas, that step has not been taken. Far more important, the failure to find excesses of soft tissue sarcomas among other workers exposed to dioxin calls into question the generality of the Swedish finding, if not the finding itself. Perhaps special conditions of exposure in Sweden contributed to their finding. Some unrecognized combination of dioxin with other chemicals or much higher levels of dioxin in Swedish herbicides (an unlikely possibility) or some other undetected peculiarity may explain this discrepancy. Regardless of what explains the Swedish findings, the conditions appear to have been present nowhere else. For example, a study of soft tissue sarcomas in New Zealand,[19] which followed the same general plan as the Swedish studies, found no case of that cancer among herbicide sprayers. Additionally, since New Zealand sprayers applied and continue to apply 2,4,5-T four months a year as compared to the two or fewer months of spraying each year in Sweden, it is reasonable to conclude that the New Zealanders were exposed to more herbicide.

Besides being present in 2,4,5-T, dioxin, as we know, is present in the chemical trichlorophenol, which is used in sawmills and in preserving animal pelts. Whereas the Swedish investigators reported an excess of soft tissue sarcoma in workers exposed to trichlorophenol, the New Zealand study found none among a comparable group of workers. The Swedish studies also revealed an excess of nasal cancers in men who worked with chlorophenol-preserved wood in sawmills and who had been exposed to dioxin in sawdust. Neither of similar studies done in Denmark and British Columbia[20] supported these results.

One fact is clear: All the Swedish case–control studies of soft tissue sarcomas and nasal cancers used the same group of people as controls.[21] What effect this might have had on the results of the studies cannot be determined, but it means, at the least, that the Swedish studies share overlapping authorship and a common control group. If there was something peculiar about the control group that exaggerated the importance of herbicide or trichlorophenol exposure in any one study, it could also have influenced the results of other studies.

Before the excesses of soft tissue sarcomas were reported, some of the same scientists who would later participate in the Swedish studies reported an excess of stomach cancers among railroad workers who had sprayed herbicides to clear rights-of-way. I am somewhat surprised that little attention has been given to this finding, because an excess of stomach cancer was also found in one population of dioxin-exposed factory workers in Germany.[22] Nevertheless, rates of the once-common stomach cancer are decreasing in Europe and the United States, and this disease may simply excite less interest than soft tissue sarcomas. More important, however, excess stomach cancers have been found in only one group of factory workers.

The Swedish studies appear to be outlyers, different from all the others, providing no convincing evidence of an association between dioxin exposure and soft tissue sarcomas; these still require confirmation. In any case, we will soon have more information about the purported association. Both the studies of Vietnam veterans by the Centers for Disease Control (CDC) and a study by the National Cancer Institute (NCI) are investigating this link further. The CDC study will not likely shed much light on this subject because of the low probability of there having been any significant exposure to dioxin in Vietnam.[23] On the other hand, the NCI study of soft tissue sarcomas in Kansas may be valuable, since a great deal of 2,4,5-T had been used there in the past. Scientists expect to publish results from this study in 1986.

Acceptance of the idea that dioxin causes soft tissue sarcomas has waxed and waned. The reports from Sweden were at first generally accepted. Perhaps the clearest evidence of this acceptance was that chemical companies and the NIOSH investigated records in the United States to see whether there were excesses of these tumors in chemical plant workers. Another indication was that the Veterans' Affairs Committees of both the House of Representatives and the Senate considered directing the Veterans Administration to compensate Vietnam veterans who developed soft tissue sarcomas. By the time they passed the compensation law, however, soft tissue sarcomas were not included, reflecting the diminished importance attached to the Swedish studies.

Contentions that dioxin causes soft tissue sarcomas evinces a common phenomenon. Once an association is suggested between dioxin exposure and any human disease or condition, the association persists even if it has little support. In particular, associations between dioxin and soft tissue sarcomas continue to be discussed although the principal authors of the Swedish papers wrote in 1984 that ". . . there is not yet any published, definite support for the Swedish epidemiologic observations."[24]

CHAPTER 14

ANIMAL TESTS OF DIOXIN TOXICITY

Let us imagine that a chemical has been present in the work-place and the environment for about 40 years. During that time, some heavily exposed chemical workers developed a persistent skin disease. But since skin diseases contracted on the job are the most often reported occupational diseases and even though the skin disease was persistent, we might decide that there was nothing exceptional about the chemical because many chemicals cause dermatitis.

Some production workers highly exposed to the chemical also displayed other signs of chemical intoxication—severe aches and pains, insomnia and irritability, liver and neurological problems. Fortunately, none of these symptoms presaged a life-threatening disease, and most subsided with time. In particular, mortality and morbidity studies found no excesses of cancer or heart disease or deaths from these causes.

Other studies of workers who had been exposed to lower amounts of the chemical showed a significant excess of a group of relatively rare cancers. Yet when other researchers tried to confirm this result in populations of similar workers around the world, the excess was found nowhere else.

A small number of pregnant women, presumably exposed to the chemical, apparently experienced a higher-than-expected rate of miscarriages, and an investigation pointed to the chemical as the cause. However, when others reexamined the design and execution of that study, they concluded that the study could not support the conclusion, and few scientists now believe it.

Repeated charges that the chemical causes birth defects have been rejected after collection and analysis of data. And, although there is no evidence for any chemical causing birth defects through exposure of the father, the Federal government launched a large and costly study to investigate the possibility that the chemical caused birth defects that way. Again, no convincing connection was found.

Finally, no one has died from acute exposure to this chemical.

In comparison to this hypothetical chemical, we know that workers heavily exposed to asbestos have twice the usual cancer rate, that cigarettes cause 100,000 cancer deaths and perhaps 120,000 heart disease deaths annually, and that alcohol is related to half the fatal automobile accidents. And still this chemical is called the most toxic chemical manufactured.

Why?

Because of its deadly effects in animal tests. It kills, causes cancer and birth defects, and damages, directly or indirectly, every organ system in laboratory animals. Of course, the "hypothetical" chemical I am referring to is dioxin.

We depend on animal tests to alert us to toxic effects. Far better, in most people's minds, to feed or inject a chemical into animals to see what amounts of it cause disease or death than to release it untested to the public and into the environment. Tests for lethal doses and skin and eye irritation, so-called "acute" effects because they are manifest soon after exposure, have been used for years and are the basis of guidance for safe handling and use of chemicals. Many objections are now raised about these tests. Some concern animal mistreatment and suffering as well as the reliability of the results as predictors of human toxicity. The results of these objections have been increased efforts to reduce the number of animals employed in tests and to develop alternative tests that do not require the use of animals.

Animal tests are also used to measure a chemical's capacity to cause cancer, birth defects, and mutations. Animal tests for these three "chronic" effects, which are not seen until some time after exposure, are held forth as providing convincing evidence of human risk by some people, but they are debated, disparaged, and dismissed by others. Debates about interpretation of animal tests often follow predictable patterns. For instance, a chemical company will probably find fault with a study that indicts one of its products as a health hazard. Animal tests for carcinogenicity, especially, become newsworthy when they show that a chemical, otherwise valuable, can cause cancer and when they are used to justify governmental regulation of a chemical. For example, in 1977, a Canadian government laboratory reported that saccharin caused bladder cancer in rats. The report created a stir that turned into a brouhaha when the United States Food and Drug Administration (FDA) sought to ban saccharin from the market. The FDA had no choice in the matter; Federal law requires it to remove ingredients from food that are shown to cause cancer in animals. The FDA was unsuccessful. Americans, unconvinced that saccharin was likely to cause cancer or willing to accept the risk to continue to enjoy a noncaloric sweetener, sent Congress an unprecedented amount of mail. Congress responded by telling the FDA to leave saccharin on the market.

So much dispute accompanies tests for carcinogenicity that it may seem that such tests are new, but as long ago as 1915, an experiment showed that rubbing rabbits' ears with soots and tars caused cancer. The experiment did not suggest anything new about the human effects of soots and tars because physicians already knew that the substances caused cancer in chimney sweeps, who were highly exposed to them. Instead, the experiment demonstrated that an animal test detected the same sort of chronic toxicity that had been seen in humans, which immediately suggested that animal testing might be the route to identify chemicals that might cause cancers in humans.

Use of animal tests for carcinogenicity was boosted immensely in the 1960s and 1970s when public concern about possible health effects from chemicals in the environment reached a fever pitch. Responding to a widespread impression that chemicals in our environment are responsible for a significant fraction of the 400,000 annual deaths from cancer in the United States,

Congress directed the National Cancer Institute (NCI) to test chemicals for their carcinogenicity.

Following a very rocky start, the NCI was never able to establish a smoothly running test system. Tests were spoiled because animals died prematurely from bacterial diseases completely unrelated to any chemical effects; other animals were killed outright by overdosing or from starvation or thirst. Moreover, results from tests that were completed went unanalyzed for months and years. Again, Congress stepped in. This time, it moved the carcinogenicity-testing program from NCI to another institute of the National Institutes of Health. Unlike all the other institutes, which are located on a university-like campus in Bethesda, Maryland, the National Institute of Environmental Health Sciences (NIEHS) is at Research Triangle Park, North Carolina. There, Congress established a new program, the National Toxicology Program (NTP), in 1979. And it is safe to say that the NTP has run the carcinogenicity-testing program like clockwork. It has also, in recent years, branched out into testing for mutations, birth defects, and neurological effects.

NTP advisory groups and government agencies nominate chemicals for testing, hold public meetings to decide where the nominated chemicals fall in a priority list, and then test the chemicals. Each cancer test costs somewhere between $500,000 and $2,000,000, uses 600 or more rats and mice, and requires 3–4 years to complete and analyze. An advisory panel, composed of representatives from academia, industry, labor, and environmental groups, reviews the results and prepares a final report stating whether or not the chemical causes cancer in animals.

Few people really care about whether a substance causes cancer in rats or mice. What everyone does care about is what the results mean for humans. So much congressional attention was given to establishing the testing program and so little to how the test results would be used that I think that it was expected that identification of a chemical as a carcinogen would be followed by reduced exposures to it, which in turn would reduce the number of cancers. The reduced exposures would be achieved through either voluntary restraints or government regulations.

It has not worked out that way. Often, exposures remain largely unchanged after the testing is done. Regulatory agencies cannot restrict exposures to hazardous chemicals with anything like the NTP's efficiency in testing them. In the absence of regulation, companies that make, use, or sell a carcinogenic chemical may act voluntarily to reduce worker exposures by installing equipment to control emissions and to contain hazardous manufacturing and disposal operations and to decrease customer exposures by reducing concentrations of the chemical in final products. However, if the chemical is economically important, the companies may attack the test's applicability for predicting human risks because it may hurt sales.

Today, it is naïve to expect manufacturers to reduce exposures automatically because some test result showed that a chemical caused cancer in animals. There is too much riding on commercial chemicals for manufacturers to acquiesce to every report that a chemical is a carcinogen. In objecting to regulation, they are sometimes supported by citizens, as in the case of saccharin.

The other flaw in expecting testing to reduce cancer was a faulty appreciation of what causes cancer. In 1979, some scientists and many members of Congress and the public said that 90% of all cancer was caused by the environment. Confusing matters was the scientists' use of the term "environment," which was different from that of other people. Scientists meant everything with which people interact, including what is eaten, smoked, drunk, and taken as medicine. Most laymen understood "the environment" to mean air, water, and soil. As part of a study that I directed at the Office of Technology Assessment (OTA), I contracted with Sir Richard Doll and Mr. Richard Peto of Oxford University, a highly esteemed epidemiologist and statistician, respectively, to compile and analyze estimates of what causes cancer. Their report[1] has become a landmark in the literature on cancer causation; its estimates have been accepted and cited repeatedly by the Department of Health and Human Services, many scientists, and the *New York Times*. Based on nationwide mortality data from 1933 through 1978, Doll and Peto estimated that 30% of all cancers were associated with smoking, about 35% with diet, 4% with industrial exposures, and 2% with exposures through air, water, and soil. The remainder they associated with viral diseases, drugs and radiation used in medicine, alcohol, and miscellaneous factors.

The estimate for the consequences of smoking is practically indisputable. Except for a few scientists who deny any connection between cigarettes and cancer, nearly all agree that upward of 100,000 people die annually from smoking-related cancers. I should note the obvious: The statistics for smoking and cancer are based on studying people, not animals.

In the spring of 1985, the OTA[2] applied Doll and Peto's method of calculating the impact of smoking to statistics from all deaths in the United States from 1978 through 1982. The OTA estimated that smoking-related cancers now account for 32% of all cancers nationwide, an increase of 2% (or 8000 additional deaths annually) over the estimate made just four years earlier. Smoking figures so prominently in causing cancer that the number of lung cancer deaths among women will exceed the number of breast cancer deaths for the first time in 1986 or 1987.

The estimate that diet is associated with 35% of all cancers has not been substantiated to anyone's satisfaction. Although people in different parts of the world who eat different diets have different cancer rates, exact relationships between foods and cancer remain to be established. It is a reasonable estimate based on what is known, and it brings attention to the undoubted importance of diet, but its accuracy is open to question. Scientists have drawn some strong statistical associations between consumption of red meat and increased colon cancer and between consumption of fiber and reduced cancer rates. However, these results are sometimes challenged because many of the studies compare cancer rates between countries, and even though Americans eat more red meat and have higher colon cancer rates than Japanese, it remains possible that other factors may be influencing cancer rates. Despite reservations about exactly how much cancer is associated with diet, the findings are already being applied. The NCI recommends that people consume less red meat and more fiber and vegetables.

Several well-known scientists attacked Doll and Peto's low

estimates for occupationally and environmentally caused cancer. Other equally well-qualified scientists greeted all the estimates with approval. Significantly, although the Doll and Peto paper was published in 1981, no review or criticism has forced significant reconsideration of their estimates.

If one accepts their estimates, as many have, then one might conclude that eliminating environmental and occupational exposures will have a relatively small effect on preventing cancer. Their estimates, to some extent, took the wind out of regulating exposures in the environment and on the job. Moreover, the Reagan administration's stated position of taking the government off the people's back through less regulation reduces the need for testing. If regulation is hardly even contemplated, little importance could be attached to gathering information to support it.

In less than two decades, the environment as a cause of cancer has reached an ascendancy and moved well back toward its starting point. The idea originated, proliferated, caused a lot of activity, and is now embattled. It would be wrong to toss it out completely. While environmental or occupational exposures do not contribute significantly to the total cancer burden they may be very important in some populations. A factory population, for instance, may be at greater risk of cancer than most people because of an occupational exposure. Recognizing that some people may be at greater risk, researchers should continue testing of chemicals for carcinogenicity and other effects as well as identifying populations more at risk. By pinpointing populations highly exposed to noxious chemicals, scientists can still make a significant contribution to health and longevity of defined populations.

Though scientists' expectations for animal tests may rise and fall, our knowledge of dioxin and our concerns about it are tied to them. The animal tests most directly related to concern about dioxin are those that measure effects at doses that produce few or no toxic effects. Neither Ranch Hands, other Vietnam veterans, the women at Alsea, nor the residents of Times Beach were made acutely ill by their exposures. They did not develop chloracne or take to bed with aches and pains or any of the other symptoms seen in industrially exposed workers or the highly exposed residents of Seveso. Still, there is concern that the long-term effects of the low exposures may result in cancer, mutations, or birth defects. These feared effects, of course, figure prominently in all discussions of environmental hazards. Congress focused on them in writing the Toxic Substances Control Act, directing the EPA to reduce exposures to substances that might cause them, and the EPA has worried about them when considering dioxin.

Before turning to tests concerned with these long-term toxicities, I will briefly review what we know about acute dioxin intoxication in animals. Tests at lethal and near-lethal doses have not revealed how dioxin kills, but they have illuminated some of its effects.

The simplest question about dioxin's toxicity may be, "How does it kill animals?" The simple answer is that we don't know. A number of biochemical changes are observed in animals that are exposed to lethal doses of dioxin, but none of these changes is sufficient to cause death.[3]

The first sign of toxicity in animals exposed to lethal or acutely toxic doses of dioxin is weight loss, including loss of adipose (fat) tissue or "wasting." The primary reason for the weight loss is reduced food consumption.[4] Dioxin alters the control mechanism that regulates food intake, so that animals end up eating too little to maintain their usual weight. Even if administration of dioxin is discontinued, the dioxin-induced change in the weight- and food-regulating mechanism persists a long time thereafter. In animals exposed to lethal doses, weight loss progresses until death occurs three weeks or more later. In some species, the rat, mouse, and guinea pig, weight loss and general debilitation can be the only symptoms before death.

Dioxin also causes degeneration of the thymus. Because this gland is important to the functioning of the immune system, several studies have looked for altered immunity in humans exposed to dioxin. Convincing evidence has not been found.[5] No relationship between dioxin exposure and reduced functioning of the immune system was found in Ranch Hands, although both smoking and advancing age profoundly depressed it.[6] Increased infectious disease frequencies, which might be expected if the immune system were significantly impaired by dioxin, have not been found. On the other hand, immune system activity increased in children exposed to dioxin at Seveso.[7] In summary, there is no convincing evidence for dioxin causing impairment of the immune system in humans. Two factors might explain these observations. Either humans are more resistant to dioxin's effects or humans have not been exposed to levels of dioxin comparable to the animal's exposures. We do not know levels of human exposure, of course, but I suspect the absence of human effects is related to lower exposures.

Although scientists have neatly cataloged dioxin's various effects on nearly every organ system in one animal or another,[8] it is a very difficult problem to sort through all the effects and come up with some common thread that will tie everything together. Alan Poland, the physician who conducted the health survey of workers at the Diamond Shamrock herbicide factory in the early 1970s,[9] has proposed a mechanism to explain dioxin's action after a decade of laboratory investigation.

Poland[10] found, in all cells that respond to dioxin, a protein that binds to molecules of dioxin as they enter the cell, forming a protein–dioxin complex. The complex then behaves like a molecular switch. It moves to a particular place on the cell's DNA, interacts with the DNA, and "turns on" a number of genes. The genes, when turned on, cause the production of a group of enzymes.

The enzymes, which are called "cytochrome P-450 enzymes" for reasons obvious to biochemists and obscure to everyone else, are a major part of the living organism's defenses against toxic chemicals. The P-450 enzymes detoxify not only man-made chemicals but also natural toxic materials, such as some toxic chemicals in plants that we eat,[11] wastes and putrefaction products in foods, and smokes from various fires. As would be expected from the variety of chemicals that we encounter as we go through life, there are many different P-450 enzymes,[12] which are turned on by different chemicals. A common name for the P-450 enzymes is "drug-metabolizing en-

zymes" because many were first discovered during drug treat-
ments and trials.

So far so good. Let us follow a molecule of dioxin after it
enters a cell. A special protein, called a "receptor protein,"
binds with the dioxin, and the receptor–dioxin complex is transported to the DNA, where it induces enzymes for the foreign
chemical's own destruction. Now the trouble begins. The induced enzymes are almost powerless against dioxin; its molecular structure making it nearly inert. Thus, it takes a long
time to eliminate dioxin from the body; up to a month is required to eliminate half the amount of ingested dioxin from the
bodies of laboratory animals.[13] An immediate consequence of
dioxin's persistence is that the enzymes stay turned on for a
long time. Although the receptor protein–dioxin complex may
come apart and fall off the DNA, if other molecules of dioxin are
present, one can interact with the receptor, form a protein–
dioxin complex, and bind again to the DNA. This process can be
repeated over and over again until the level of dioxin at last falls
below some critical level.

Outside of tying up a part of the cell's metabolic machinery,
continued production of P-450 enzymes seems to have no toxic
effect. However, cells that are damaged by dioxin, such as those
in the thymus, are thought to have in addition a second group of
genes that can also be turned on, and the enzyme products of
the second group of genes damage the cells. Poland, who proposed this idea, has no information about whether the dioxin-
receptor complex that turns on the P-450 enzymes also turns on
the toxic genes or whether some product from P-450 enzyme
activity turns on the second group of genes.

A reasonable question is why do any cells have toxic genes.
There is no clear answer to this question yet. Poland thinks that
they are genes for controlling cellular proliferation that are normally turned off, but are turned on in response to such unusual
toxic chemicals as dioxin. Since dioxin is persistent in the cell,
the genes for the toxic enzymes will remain turned on for a long
time.

This model neatly explains why a receptor protein is necessary for dioxin's toxicity, why the P-450 enzymes are turned on

in all cells that have a receptor complex, and why toxic effects are not detectable in all these cells. Toxic effects are limited to those cells in which toxic enzymes are produced.

Scientists have partially purified the receptor protein, so we know that it exists. They also know that the dioxin–receptor complex binds to DNA and that neither dioxin nor the receptor by itself does. Furthermore, from all they know about interactions between receptor complexes and DNA, when the receptor falls off the DNA, the DNA remains unchanged by the interaction. These facts are critically important to understanding the mechanisms by which dioxin might cause mutations, cancer, and birth defects.

Mutations, which are changes in the structure of DNA, can cause permanent changes in a cell's biology. The best-understood mutagen (i.e., agent that causes mutations) is radiation of various kinds. At doses well below those necessary to cause overt toxicity, radiation can inactivate a gene, alter a gene's functioning, or cause rearrangements in DNA. When the mutation occurs in a germ cell—an egg cell or a sperm cell—it causes no observable effect at all in the animal in which it occurs. However, if a mutated egg is fertilized or a mutated sperm fertilizes an egg cell during reproduction, every cell of the new organism will bear a copy of the mutation, with sometimes devastating effects.

Mutations that occur in somatic cells are not passed on to the next generation (all the cells in the body except for the sex cells—sperm in men, ova in women—are called "somatic cells"). Some somatic mutations simply kill the cell in which they occur, which is a trivial event. Organs and tissues have millions or billions of cells, and death and replenishment are common. More serious are somatic mutations that set in motion a train of events that can result in cancer, and many carcinogens (agents that cause cancer) also cause mutations.

Because of the profound effects of mutagens on the health of the next generation and in cancer causation, a great number of chemical and biological tests have been developed to assay for mutagenic activity. Scattered among hundreds of published reports are a few that conclude that dioxin is a mutagen. On balance, the evidence for this conclusion is quite weak, and many of the positive reports are directly contradicted by results from other laboratories. The NTP found that dioxin did not cause mutations in a battery of standard tests, underscoring its lack of mutagenic activity.[14]

Another serious objection to the idea that dioxin is a mutagen comes from chemical experiments that measured its affinity for DNA. Mutagens (and some, if not all, carcinogens) interact physically and chemically with DNA, binding to it and altering its structure. Dioxin binds to DNA 10,000–1,000,000 times less avidly than do known mutagens and carcinogens.[15]

Both its limited biological activity in tests for mutagenicity and its minimal chemical interactions with DNA lead to the conclusion that dioxin is not an active mutagen. This finding not only predicts that dioxin does not cause mutations, but also influences how we think about dioxin as a cause of cancer.

There is no doubt that dioxin causes cancer in laboratory animals. The NTP tested dioxin to see whether it causes cancer when applied to the backs of mice. It did,[16] but the resulting tumors were the same type that are caused by inserting inert plastic pellets into mouse skin.[17] The pellets do not cause cancer by interacting with DNA; instead, the cancers appear to arise as a growth response to irritation. Because dioxin does not interact with DNA and because of the kind of skin cancer caused by it, it is probable that the skin cancers caused by dioxin arose from a mechanism similar to that of the inert plastic pellets. In other words, the dioxin applied to the mouse's back is not behaving "chemically" at all; instead, it is a physical irritant.

Two well-conducted experiments have shown that ingested dioxin causes liver and thyroid cancer in rats and mice. One of the tests, which involved administration of dioxin through a stomach tube (by "gavage"), a routine method, was done by Federal scientists.[18] The other, which involved feeding dioxin mixed in the animals' food, was done by Dow scientists.[19] Both the Federal scientists and the Dow scientists fully described their experiments and results, which are quite similar, and both experiments are accepted by the scientific community as equally good. The Dow study has been considered more useful for making predictions about human risks, however, because it was somewhat larger.[20]

Not all animals exposed to cancer-causing doses of dioxin actually developed cancer, but microscopic examination of the livers of all animals exposed to these doses revealed extensive tissue damage. Moreover, the animals were made visibly ill by their continuous two-year-long exposure. The tissue damage probably resulted from dioxin causing continual production of the cytochrome P-450 enzymes and possibly toxic enzymes. Researchers also observed the same kind of damage in some animals exposed to lower doses of dioxin, which further supports the idea that dioxin-caused cancer occurs most often following significant tissue damage. Less has been published about changes in the thyroid, the other organ in which dioxin causes cancer. However, dioxin causes detectable changes in this organ, and some evidence that dioxin's interaction with the thyroid is important to the chemical's lethality.[21] Therefore, tissue damage or at least biochemical alteration of both the liver and thyroid often accompanies dioxin's causing cancer therein.

Cancer causation is thought to involve at least two complicated and complex steps—initiation and promotion. Initiation is seen as a mutational event that permanently changes the DNA of a cell. Scientists consider it a "clean" event, meaning it is not necessarily accompanied by any detectable toxic effects. Promotion is an event or sequence of events, subsequent to initiation, that promotes the growth and multiplication of the mutant cells. Promotion, on the other hand, is not "clean" and is marked by observable toxic effects. These definitions are somewhat vague, but they are all we have.[22]

Although not every scientist accepts every detail of the initiator–promoter sequence, almost all agree that the progression from normal to cancerous growth has more than one step and that the first step is a mutational event. The first step is also called "genotoxic," because it inflicts damage on DNA, the genetic material. Since dioxin neither binds to DNA nor causes mutations, it is not genotoxic and has no demonstrable initiator properties. By the process of elimination, if the initiator–promoter idea has any validity, dioxin should be a promoter.

Typical of promoters is the detectable tissue damage of the sort observed in the livers of rats and mice exposed to quantities of dioxin sufficient to cause cancer. More to the point, Poland and his colleagues have demonstrated that dioxin is a promoter of cancer in mouse skin[23] and rat liver.[24]

How, then, can we explain the fact that dioxin has caused tumors when it was the only toxic chemical fed to laboratory animals? It may be that something in the food of the animals served as an initiator or that the toxic doses of dioxin used in these tests behaved as both initiator and promoter.

Discussion of dioxin's capacity to cause cancer is complicated because the words "low dose" and "high dose" become confusing. Dioxin, by whatever mechanism, caused cancer in animals at a lower absolute dose than any other chemical tested by the NTP. Nevertheless, its carcinogenicity appears to differ in degree and not in kind from that of its chemical relatives, the chlorinated hydrocarbons; all cause liver and thyroid cancers in animals. In addition, while dioxin is extremely carcinogenic, it is also exceedingly toxic, causing extensive damage in the organs in which it causes cancer. A group of researchers at Harvard has analyzed a mass of data and find that, in general, the more toxic a chemical is, the more carcinogenic it is, and that dioxin's ratio of toxicity to carcinogenicity parallels the ratio for many other chemicals. Moreover, dioxin is no more carcinogenic than would be predicted from its toxicity.[25] Therefore, the carcinogenic dose is "high" in the sense that it causes overt toxicity. Even doses 1/10th as great as those that cause cancer cause some detectable liver toxicity.

What this means for human risk is not entirely clear, but if dioxin causes cancer only at toxic doses, it suggests that human cancer risks from dioxin are quite low. Few humans have ever been exposed to doses that affected liver function, and even those that have been have suffered no excess of cancer.

Tests that showed dioxin causes birth defects alarmed scientists and citizens about dioxin's threat to health. In these tests, 2,4,5-T administered to pregnant mice caused cleft palates and kidney abnormalities in their newborn pups. Follow-up investigations showed that it was not the 2,4,5-T itself, but the dioxin it contained, that caused the birth defects. Since these first experiments, pregnant mice, rats, rabbits, monkeys, and other animals have been exposed to dioxin.

In some but not all experiments, a tiny dose (1 microgram dioxin/kilogram body weight) administered each day to a pregnant mouse was sufficient to cause a measurable increase in cleft palates. A dose three times higher caused cleft palate in all experiments, but it also caused fetal death and maternal toxicity. In animals other than mice, dioxin caused fetal deaths but not birth defects, emphasizing again that the chemical's effects differ from species to species. However, maternal toxicity was commonly observed at the same doses that caused fetal death.

Though minuscule amounts have caused cleft palates in mice, it is almost impossible for humans to consume proportionally that much. Some Australian scientists have calculated the proportional dose for a 110-pound woman. She would have to ingest a half ounce or more of dioxin-containing 2,4,5-T per day. If the source of 2,4,5-T was meat from animals that had grazed on sprayed vegetation, she would have to consume between 13,200 and 198,000 pounds of meat daily or drink 3975 to 238,000 gallons of sprayed water daily to take in an amount of dioxin equivalent to the amount that caused birth defects in mice.[26]

Thus, the results of animal tests for teratogenicity (the capacity to cause birth defects) leave us in much the same quandry as the animal tests for cancer. The effects are seen only at exposure levels that cause overt toxicity. I know of no claims of maternal toxicity from dioxin in women, and if such toxicity accompanies doses necessary for birth defects, such exposures must be exceedingly rare.

To allow for the possibility that humans are more sensitive than the most sensitive test animal, scientists often determine the lowest dose necessary to cause birth defects in a laboratory animal and then apply a "safety factor." For instance, if 1 microgram of dioxin per kilogram body weight in mice causes no effect, then a dose 1000 times smaller will be proposed as a safe dose in humans. If we apply such a safety factor to the calculation mentioned above of the Australian scientists, a woman would have to consume between 13 and 198 pounds of dioxin-contaminated meat or drink between 4 and 238 gallons of contaminated water daily to exceed a safe level.

Pregnant monkeys are especially sensitive to continual exposure to dioxin. Although the exposures do not cause birth defects, they do cause spontaneous abortions, accompanied by maternal toxicity. If pregnant women resemble pregnant female monkeys in their sensitivity to dioxin, a pregnant woman would have to consume about 30,000 pounds of meat containing the highest reported levels of dioxin daily for a week to accumulate a dose of dioxin equivalent to the one that caused spontaneous abortions in monkeys. If a woman were to consume dioxin-contaminated meat continuously throughout her lifetime, she would have to eat 250 pounds of the dioxin-containing meat a day to accumulate an amount of dioxin equivalent to that which caused an increased risk of miscarriage in monkeys.[27] We do not know how closely the biology of humans and monkeys is related, but we should consider taking some comfort from the fact that abortions in monkeys occur only at near toxic doses, far greater than amounts of dioxin that any woman ever encountered.

Exposing either males or females to dioxin before mating does not cause birth defects. These results are clear and offer no support for the idea that exposures prior to mating cause risk to the next generation. Of course, people who are convinced that dioxin causes birth defects can argue that the animal tests were not done correctly and that if they were, effects would be found. To respond to these contentions with another test would not necessarily settle the question. If the additional tests found no effects, the argument could be made again that the tests were wrong. As we have seen repeatedly, it is impossible to prove a negative.

What does all this mean for humans? It would be very reassuring to conclude that dioxin, at worst, causes cancer and fetal death only at toxic or very nearly toxic doses. We know now that chemical workers who were made sick by dioxin have no elevated cancer rates. Since they do not, if overt toxicity is a prerequisite for carcinogenicity, it might be reasonable to think that people exposed to levels of dioxin that cause no overt symptoms are at no elevated risk of cancer or birth defects.

However, it may not be so simple. In an animal test for cancer, scientists examine about 100 animals at each dose level. Therefore, they cannot detect cancers that occur less frequently than 1 in 100 animals. If the dose caused cancer in only 1 of 200 animals, that effect would go undetected. To allow for the possibility that a chemical causes cancer at frequencies that are undetectable in practical tests, government regulatory agencies assume that some level of risk is associated with all doses above zero, with the risk increasing with increasing dose. For instance, the EPA sets exposure limits so that no person who is exposed to that amount of a carcinogenic chemical has greater than a one in a million risk of developing cancer. To estimate that limit, the EPA determines the smallest amount of a chemical that causes cancer. Let us say that a dose of 1 microgram of dioxin per kilogram body weight per day causes cancer in 50% of the exposed animals. As an approximation, we can divide that dose by one million to estimate the acceptable daily dose for humans over a lifetime.

I think this can be a reasonable approach for chemicals that act as initiators. Once a mutation is caused in DNA, it remains there, ready to progress to a cancer if the right promoters come along. I do not think that simply dividing the smallest dose that causes cancer in animals by a million is appropriate for promoters, however. Along with many scientists,[28] I think that higher exposure levels are acceptable for promoters. Although there is no generally accepted method for estimating a safe level for promoters, one method that is often mentioned is to apply a "safety factor" to the dose that causes cancer in animals. When this is done for dioxin, the daily dose of dioxin that would be so low as not to cause cancer is about the same as doses calculated to be sufficiently low not to cause birth defects or spontaneous abortions in humans.

Dioxin is the most toxic manufactured chemical (except for some chemical warfare agents), and it is the most potent carcinogen tested by the Federal government. Despite its toxicity, it has not killed any human being. Furthermore, it causes cancer in animals only at near-toxic or toxic doses, and it has not been shown to increase human cancer rates even in people who were made sick by it. It also causes birth defects (in mice only) and spontaneous abortions at doses that cause overt toxicity. In other words, cancer, birth defects, and spontaneous abortions are seen only at (or very near) exposure levels that cause visible illness within a few days or weeks of exposure. Does that mean humans are not at risk if they are not made ill by dioxin exposure? Not necessarily. If, indeed, there is some risk at any dose, human risk may be present at exceedingly low doses. So far, the absence of convincing evidence for human cancer, birth defects, and spontaneous abortions does not bear out the idea that it presents a risk at these tiny doses.

Risk remains an unmeasurable quality; it is made up of estimates. Although studies of human populations can measure the harm that dioxin may have caused, they can provide no resolution about the level of risk associated with dioxin. For instance, epidemiological studies generally cannot reliably detect increases in cancer rates that are less than a doubling. Although no doubling of cancer has been seen in people exposed to dioxin, human studies cannot rule out a smaller increase.

Hundreds of animal studies have alerted us to dioxin's risk for humans, but epidemiology has yet to demonstrate that it has harmed humans except to cause chloracne and some transient effects in highly exposed workers. The American Medical Association has little to gain, one way or the other, from deciding or not deciding that dioxin has harmed or is likely to harm humans. Its Council on Scientific Affairs[29] concluded in 1984:

> Adverse reactions [from dioxin] in animals include . . . [degeneration of the thymus, induction of liver enzymes, birth defects in mice, and spontaneous abortions in rodents and monkeys]. Except for chloracne, however, TCDD [dioxin] has not demonstrated comparable levels of biologic activity in man; that is to say, no long-term effects on the cardiovascular and central nervous systems, the liver, the kidney, the thymus and immunologic defenses, and the

reproductive function—in the male, female or offspring—
have been demonstrated.

We are left with a quandary. The absence of detectable harm in exposed people has reduced the level of concern about dioxin. On the other hand, high estimates of cancer risk derived from the EPA's and other agencies' extrapolations of risk from animal tests still maintain the level of concern about environmental exposures higher than is justified. The extrapolations are based on what many scientists widely perceive to be misinterpretations of the mechanism by which dioxin causes cancer.

CHAPTER 15

DIOXIN DECISIONS

The picture I paint contrasts sharply with the popular depiction of dioxin as a scourge to human health. How can two views of the same thing differ so much? Is there any chance that the two views will come closer in perspective to each other?

The latter question is easier to answer, and my response would be yes as the dioxin controversy recedes from public attention. In recent coverage, the *New York Times* has printed relatively low-key descriptions of dioxin referring to it as "a potentially carcinogenic substance"[1] in one article and as "a hazardous substance"[2] in another. In editorials on the Agent Orange trial, the *Times* agreed with the judge who declared that no connection was shown between use of that herbicide and health effects in veterans.[3] Eventually, such balanced reporting of dioxin's effects will chip away if not blot out altogether dioxin's reputation as the "most toxic manufactured chemical."

In three celebrated court cases, the judge or the jury had to decide about dioxin's effects on humans. The three judgments agree that dioxin has caused no detectable long-term or life-threatening human harm. As mentioned earlier, the judge in the Nova Scotia case pronounced that plaintiffs who had sought to stop use of pesticides containing dioxin had failed to prove "any strong probability or a sufficient degree of probability of risk to health"[4] from such use and ruled that its use could continue. In the well-publicized Agent Orange trial, the judge concluded that the veterans were unable to prove that any of the illnesses and birth defects they claimed to result from dioxin had actually been caused by it. In the Monsanto trial, the jury found that the effects of dioxin were not "life-threatening."

Nonetheless, courts are generally considered a poor place to decide scientific questions; only the rare judge or juror has technical training to make an informed judgment. Because of their technical limitations and reliance on human experience, evidence, and emotion, juries would seem more likely than scientists to focus on the plantiffs' illnesses rather than on what caused them. To offset bias introduced by human nature, both sides in the court cases introduced expert witnesses. Spelling out assumptions about biological relationships between mice and men, the scientist as an expert witness would likely say that dioxin at some very low level may increase the risk of cancer by one in a million; at 100 times that dosage, the risk is increased to one in 10,000 or 100 in a million and so forth. The emergence of risk analysis in the courtroom—the presenting of potential hazards in statistical terms—is a relatively new phenomenon. Other expert witnesses may present, explain, and interpret the studies of possible associations between dioxin and human harm. While all this information might overwhelm judges and juries, the courts, in the aforementioned three most celebrated cases, have assimilated and used it.

Courts, in civil suits, rely on evidence and expert witnesses to demonstrate that a preponderance of the evidence favors a particular side. Often, that decision hangs on the two words "but for." Would the person who claims damage have escaped that damage *but for* his or her exposure to dioxin? It is a difficult thing to weigh a one-in-a-million risk derived from animal studies in making that decision. Moreover, scientists draw attention to the uncertainty of their data and extrapolation methods, testifying that the risk estimates could be off by a factor of 10 or 100 or more, which to some extent undercuts the usefulness of their information. I think, therefore, that such difficulties largely negate reliance on animal studies in the courts' decision-making, although the evidence is certainly heard and discussed.

The absence of pertinent, specific facts concerning the exact amounts of exposure also plagues the courts. At Nitro, many workers were afflicted with chloracne, indicating high exposure levels. Since no one developed chloracne after being exposed to spraying with 2,4,5-T in forests or with Agent Orange in Vietnam, lower exposure levels are indicated in these situations. But when it comes to quantitative specifics, there remain only question marks. We do not know whether the high exposures that caused chloracne are twice as high as the lower ones, 10 times higher, 100 times higher, or even more. Equally important, we do not know how many micrograms or milligrams of dioxin anyone was exposed to. Without that basic knowledge, we cannot predict how many excess cases of disease would be expected in the exposed populations, even if we take the extrapolated risk factors from animal studies at face value.

Now we come, I think, to the crux of the difference between estimated risk and measured harm. A person who claims harm from dioxin can point to his or her affliction as evidence of injury, but how does he or she prove that dioxin actually caused it? Animal studies show that it is possible, but that is all they can show. The injured person has only limited human evidence to show that dioxin causes effects in humans. In none of the three court cases did the scanty and disputed human data showing that dioxin caused adverse effects support the claim that "but for" the exposure to dioxin the injured persons would have been well. No disease has dioxin as its unique cause; even chloracne can be caused by related chemicals. The same dreadful afflictions that affect those who have been exposed to dioxin strike others who have never been near it. Furthermore, studies of dioxin-exposed populations have failed to produce convincing evidence of excesses of disease.

The lack of proof for human harm does not mean that the levels of risk extrapolated from animal studies are wrong. Epidemiology simply cannot provide information about small risks.

I expect that the judgments in the Nova Scotia, Agent Orange, and Monsanto cases, all within a two-year period, will slow any flood of dioxin litigation. The diminished legal activity will contribute to a general impression of a lessening of disputes about dioxin's effects. There being fewer trials, there will be fewer opportunities for television discussions and debates between lawyers or experts from each side. Although these discussions are educational, they often highlight extreme positions and seldom offer the viewer guidance as to which of the opposing views is generally accepted as more credible by scientists.

Often forgotten in the furor about dioxin, 2,4,5-T is no longer produced in the United States, and little of its precursor, trichlorophenol, is being manufactured. These facts are of paramount importance, since according to the EPA,[5] nearly every finding of dioxin in the environment has been associated with trichlorophenol's production or disposal. Certain risks surround every landfill and every barrel of trichlorophenol and 2,4,5-T wastes buried around the country, but to the extent that these chemicals threaten human health, the risk has been greatly reduced since the 1960s, when 15 million pounds of 2,4,5-T were produced annually. Since 1980, Federal regulations have required that companies that dispose of any materials containing dioxin or any materials or machinery ever used in the manufacture of trichlorophenol must notify the EPA of the disposal. Moreover, the waste must be transported to an approved disposal site. I do not pretend that notification is complete or that approved disposal sites are necessarily secure[6] (it is a tricky thing to be sure that dumps will not leak and even trickier to find an insurance company that will provide a policy against liability if they do leak), but these requirements have surely further reduced risks.

The question before the courts in the Agent Orange and Monsanto cases was one of compensation. Congress has also considered compensation for veterans who claim damage from Agent Orange. In 1984, Congress directed the Veterans Administration (VA) to compensate Vietnam veterans for cases of chloracne or porphyria cutanea tarda (the rare skin and liver disease) if either appeared within one year of a veteran's leaving Southeast Asia. From a scientific standpoint, the association between dioxin and chloracne is indisputable, but that between dioxin and porphyria cutanea tarda is highly questionable.[7] Congress, however, responded to veterans' desires for compensation by treating both the same in passing that law. Just as these diseases are rare among the population at large, there are essentially no reports of them among veterans.

The fact that the law has and will compensate no more than a handful of veterans for these rare diseases does not represent false stewardship on the part of Congress. Congress, unsure whether anyone had been exposed to sufficient quantities of dioxin to cause disease, provided compensation in case anyone had been.

Congress considered other diseases for compensation, soft tissue sarcomas being the most commonly mentioned. I think, without much evidence, that Congress discounted the evidence from studies of Swedish lumberjacks that showed an excess of these cancers resulting from herbicide exposures when other studies from around the world failed to confirm them. Whether or not this is the reason, the decision not to include soft tissue sarcomas reflects a pulling back from presumptions that Agent Orange causes life-threatening diseases, which in turn reflects less support for the idea that exposures to dioxin in the environment have caused adverse health effects.

Congress passed no law establishing compensation for birth defects in veterans' children, although such legislation was considered. The birth defects study by the Centers for Disease Control (CDC) caused a flurry of activity when it reported excesses of spina bifida, cleft lip, and neoplasms among children born to veterans who might have been exposed to Agent Orange. Bills were drafted and discussed privately, but went no further. I think that the CDC's careful discussion of the possible meaning of the results of its study and its authors' in-person explanations to Congress—that the reported excesses did not prove or even offer much support for an association between Agent Orange exposure and birth defects—convinced Congress not to continue with compensation legislation. The CDC scientists contended that there was no biological explanation for dioxin causing birth defects through exposure of the father, that the estimates of Agent Orange exposure were flawed, and that the reported associations might have been due to chance.[8]

The court and Congressional decisions suggest that the perception of dioxin's effect on humans is slipping from a much-discussed great hazard to a less-discussed, smaller one. The division between those convinced that dioxin causes dreadful diseases and those who view its effects as minor will persist. It will not change. But voices in the former camp are not increasing in number, while scientists who have not voiced an opinion before are joining the latter. As opportunities to expound on dioxin's toxicity diminish because of fewer publicized court cases and congressional actions, it may appear that some common ground between the two extremes is being reached. I doubt that agreements will be reached; instead, the arguments will disappear from public view.

Although television airings reporting trials will diminish, the completion of government studies about dioxin will garner news coverage. I expect that the studies will be largely or completely negative, finding few or no associations between dioxin exposure and disease or death. It is probable that as each report is released, the principal investigator will be interviewed, state his or her conclusions, and be shunted off-camera and replaced by a proponent of the view that dioxin has caused many adverse health effects. The proponent will likely disagree with the study results, saying that the study was incompetently done or biased, but be able to offer no evidence that the flaws, if any, are responsible for the negative results. Instead, the proponent may be limited to opinions or impressions that something important has been overlooked or ignored, and he or she may be right. Nonetheless, the news madia, in making such "balanced" presentations, project anecdotal accounts as somehow equal in structure and validity to large, well-conducted studies. In leaving the viewer to choose between the negative study and the proponent's views, it obscures the emerging consensus about the absence of demonstrable effects of dioxin on human health and, I think, downgrades the contributions of scientists who conduct honest, credible studies.

Whatever technical debates continue to rage, nonpartisans in the dioxin debate will come to accept, I think, the judgments of courts and Congress that the case for human effects remains unproved, and as the hubbub diminishes, they will realize that it is unprovable. Eventually, the disagreements will fade from view, leaving the widely variant estimates of dioxin's risk unreconciled but of little importance to public policy.

Still, how can the various estimates of dioxin's risks vary so much? The expression "Bad things happen to good people" sums up events that cannot be ignored. Apparently healthy women in Alsea could not carry babies to term, and veterans, returning from Vietnam, fell prey to various diseases. It is human nature to ask why such things occur. Long ago, evil spirits caused disease and misfortune; at times in history, witches cast spells. Now we look for physical causes, and our life-spans have increased as causes of disease have been pinpointed and controlled. When confronted with an unexpected disease today and when we have little or no information about its cause, we often point to the environment, specifically chemicals in the environment, as the culprit.

The idea of an environmental cause for a disease is very seductive. First, it provides a reason for the misfortune. Moreover, it absolves the harmed person from sharing or bearing responsibility for the misfortune and confers responsibility for controlling the misfortune on someone else. Of the two, the first reason is most important, in part because identification of cause is the first step to control.

Once a connection is made between an environmental factor and disaster, individuals and organizations will begin publicizing it. Naturally, they will want to alert other people of a potential danger, in itself, a praiseworthy deed. In some cases, however, whistle blowers, without meaning to, seriously distort the facts. For instance, in late 1983, an envelope with DIOXIN printed large across its face dropped through my front-door mail slot. The letter inside urged me to join the Environmental Defense Fund (EDF), promising that my membership money would help ". . . spread the whole truth about dioxin." The letter listed every charge ever leveled against dioxin, blasted Dow for having known about dioxin's "health risks as early as 1965," and castigated Dow for mounting a publicity campaign that said "Dioxin poses no serious threat to human health" at the same time the company was a defendant in the Agent Orange trial. The EDF did not say that the human health effects of dioxin are far from agreed on, that the effect Dow knew about in 1965 was chloracne—never a concern from environmental

exposures—or why Dow's conducting a publicity campaign
while it was in court was offensive. This letter was mailed to
more than 350,000 addresses. To the extent that it was read, it
contributed to the impression that dioxin has had a devastating
effect on human health.

On the other end of the spectrum are proponents who contend that dioxin in 2,4,5-T presents no risk. Dioxin may have
caused little convincing, demonstrated harm, but it is still a risk.
Congress and the regulatory agencies have already established
in the case of dioxin as well as other chemicals that a one-in-a-
million lifetime risk of cancer is sufficient to justify regulatory
action. Though this risk is unequivocally small, and though current risks from environmental exposures to dioxin may be even
smaller, it is not analogous to "no risk."

In addition to civil law courts, administrative law courts
have heard dioxin cases. Administrative law courts decide
whether or not regulations restricting manufacture, use, and
disposal of hazardous chemicals are justified to protect the public health. There is no contradiction between civil courts finding
dioxin not guilty of causing human harm and administrative law
courts deciding that stringent regulations are necessary to protect public health from the risks of dioxin. The laws that regulate
chemical exposures—the Toxic Substances Control Act, the
Federal Insecticide, Fungicide, and Rodenticide Act, and the
Food, Drug, and Cosmetics Act—are designed to reduce risks.
They specifically allow or require that animal test results be
considered in deciding whether a chemical poses a risk. In regulations written under these laws, the inability of epidemiology
or any other method to disprove a one-in-a-million or a one-in-
ten-thousand risk leaves the animal data unassailable as an estimate of risk. In civil courts, these risk estimates would take a
back seat to questions about whether or not harm had been
done.

Some scientists interpret the data from animal studies on
dioxin to mean that the chemical is capable of causing significant
human harm. Many of these scientists, who work for or volunteer their services to environmental organizations, do not have
financial resources at their disposal to support new animal test-

ing programs or epidemiological studies. It takes no more than a minute to figure out that Dow can and the EDF cannot. However, if scientists affiliated with environmental organizations cannot undertake new research, they can review the available data and present their analyses, interpretations, and opinions at scientific meetings and by writing letters to science journals.

An editorial[9] in *Science*—one of the most prestigious scientific journals—said that the health risks of dioxin were exaggerated. A letter of rebuttal followed, providing an example of a scientist bringing to the attention of other scientists literature that supports his view. The letter[10] refers to a paper about the Seveso explosion and claims large increases in abortions and birth defects, but does not mention that these data are considered unreliable because of ignorance of the rates of these problems before the explosion and difficulties in measuring rates afterward. The letter blames scientists employed by industry who analyzed mortality data among factory workers for having missed an increase in "soft tissue carcinomas and lymphomas." While it is true that National Institute for Occupational Safety and Health (NIOSH) scientists, not industry scientists, combined information from a number of studies and reports of soft tissue sarcoma cases to determine the total number of reported cases in the chemical industry, the initial reports of these cases were made by industry scientists. In any case, subsequent reanalysis of the same data reduced the number of soft tissue sarcomas among workers exposed to dioxin from seven to two. The NIOSH has been unable to decide whether this is more than the expected number because it is uncertain about the actual rate of occurrence of these tumors in chemical workers and in the general population.[11]

The same letter also makes reference to reported increases in liver cancer, spontaneous abortions, stillbirths, and malformed children among Vietnamese exposed to Agent Orange. The increase in liver cancer rates reported by a Vietnamese scientist in 1973 during the Vietnam War has not been supported by any other study. The increase in reproductive problems was reported by Vietnamese scientists at meetings or in journals that do not send papers out for review by other scientists. This is not a fatal flaw, but until the methodology of the studies is reviewed by other knowledgeable scientists, the conclusions should be considered tentative. I do not automatically discredit studies done by Vietnam scientists. I know, for instance, that the Pasteur Institute in Hanoi has long been an active research center for capable scientists. However, the ability to do credible epidemiology in a country with poor records that is still emerging from a devastating war, strains my credulity. My reaction to these studies is colored by the knowledge that Guinness's book of records lists the longest life-spans in countries with the highest illiteracy rates. Without records, any epidemiology study depends on recall, and recall can be faulty.

The letter, probably read by thousands of scientists, provides references to the literature that support the writer's viewpoint. The reader of *Science* who has not followed the dioxin debate might take these references as a reflection of all that is known about dioxin's health effects. The more knowledgeable reader would realize that an abundant amount of literature was neglected.

A year and a half later, a letter appeared in *Nature*,[12] the highly respected British science journal. It cites two publications in *Science* as evidence in the controversy about dioxin's health effects. A reader of the *Nature* letter who did not check the references would probably assume that the references were to research articles. However, they were not; they were to the *Science* editorial and letter of rebuttal.

The *Nature* letter commented on the two mortality studies done at the Monsanto plant in Nitro. It did not directly disagree with the conclusions reached in those papers that dioxin has not caused an excess of cancer or early death, but it highlighted the lamentable gaffe that four men who died from cancer were classified as exposed in one paper and unexposed in the other. Although the differing classifications are disquieting, three of the deaths were from lung cancer, never associated with dioxin, and the other from Hodgkin's disease, for which there is little evidence of association with dioxin. The contradictory classifications were not covered up in the original papers; they were simply overlooked. Moreover, because the results were published in the open scientific literature, other scientists had the opportunity to discover the errors.

The *Nature* letter also states that 19 workers who died from cancer or cardiovascular disease were not included in either mortality study, suggesting an oversight or coverup. However, if the 19 left Monsanto before 1955, they would have been excluded from one study because the company had only incomplete records on men who left the company prior to that time, and from the other study if they had not been present at the 1949 explosion. Again, a deficiency in the study is evident, but not anything necessarily sinister.

After identifying flaws in the mortality studies, the letter makes a plea for reexamination of all the data from Nitro. No one can object to that. However, the letter itself was not from neutral observers. Both authors had testified for the plaintiffs in the Nitro trial, but neither they nor *Nature* mentions that they had.

Many scientists, just like many people in every other walk of life, are interested in the topic of dioxin; only a minority, however, have familiarized themselves with the plethora of available literature. The controversy, though somewhat muted, remains. One of the factors contributing to the polemic is that various scientists draw attention to different data in order to make their points. Another factor, as in any debate, is that statements and questions can be posed differently by the two sides.

For example, some Vietnam veterans and a few scientists assert that Agent Orange causes cancer, and other scientists firmly hold that there is no evidence to support this claim. But they are not addressing themselves to the same point. Veterans and their supporters claim that dioxin is a carcinogen; the others state that there is no evidence for carcinogenicity in humans. The doubters do not say that dioxin is definitely not a carcinogen, only that there is no evidence for its causing cancer in humans. A single convincing positive study, showing that dioxin is associated with increased human cancer, could lead scientists to conclude that the chemical is a human carcinogen. Scientists, in their fashion, review existing literature and replow already-worked fields on the chance that something has been overlooked. As the studies go on, people who do not accept the evidence already available can say the "jury is still out" on dioxin's health effects. Paradoxically, in real courtrooms, judges and juries have already made their decisions.

Society is traveling on two tracks. Congress, judges, and juries have evaluated the available evidence, made decisions, and assigned responsibilities. Science, on the other hand, continues to do its studies. I expect that the results from scientific studies will become of little more than academic interest unless they find overwhelming evidence of human damage. By the time results are available, many of the important decisions will have been made. A number have already been made.

Many of my fellow scientists think that courts should make no decisions about technical issues. The courts have little choice, of course. When cases are brought before them, they have a responsibility to decide them, and their decisions are made in the context of the times. The Agent Orange trial had its origins in a divisive war—it had emotional, social, and political overtones. The judge in that case, who read all the technical information, concluded that there was no proof that human harm had been shown. In his opinion, a jury, despite having great sympathy for the afflicted veterans, would have weighed the evidence about harm and found it lacking. The Monsanto jury made some observations about dioxin's limited health effects, but its legal importance was its statement that Monsanto had not been negligent of its workers' health given the standards of the 1940s and 1950s. The Nova Scotia case, however, was more narrowly based on evidence about risk. Since no one could show that he or she had been harmed by dioxin-contaminated herbicides or that he or she was likely to be, the judge allowed the continued spraying of forests.

No matter what additional information becomes available, dioxin and Agent Orange have been incorporated into the nation's store of common knowledge. A humorous piece in *The New Yorker*[13] made Agent Orange the ultimate weapon against the spread of "Japanese knotweed . . . known to botanists as the cockroach of the vegetable kingdom." In 1983, at the time Ann Burford was deciding to resign as Administrator of the EPA, a parody of the song "Hard-Hearted Anna" was presented at my neighborhood's annual musical review. One line, "Dioxin, the toxin, the stuff you wash your socks in," reflected concern about the chemical's wide dissemination in the environment. Far more seriously, a mystery novel blames a veteran's deviant behavior on dioxin. After the veteran, a nephew of a hard-boiled private detective, dies hanging from a tree in southern Iowa, the detective's investigation reveals that the veteran has lived in a cave, farmed marijuana for a living, and been a general nuisance. While serving in Vietnam, he had killed dozens of people—enemies, "friendlies," and at least one American officer—on orders. The detective concludes that regardless of what these experiences might have done to the veteran's psyche: "Billy [the veteran] was sick. I'm not positive, but I think he was poisoned by something called Agent Orange, a defoliant they used over in Vietnam."[14] Clive Cussler's novel *Deep Six*[15] is about a mysterious chemical that almost instantly kills any animal that comes in contact with it. One of Cussler's heroes says that the chemical threatens "all marine life in the Gulf of Alaska" and if it is carried south, "could poison every man, fish, animal, and bird as far away as Mexico." Although at the time he did not know the identity of the substance, he is able to narrow his choices: "The three worst poisonous substances known to man are plutonium, dioxin and a chemical warfare system." The last turns out to be the culprit in the story, but dioxin has certainly achieved literary notoriety.

In the real world, the most certain thing is that a number of studies about possible health effects will be completed in the next few years. If any reveals a significant health threat, everything will change. Congress will act, and courts may hear about "2,4-D and 2,4,5-T," "chloracne and soft tissue sarcomas" again. Clearly, I am betting against that.

If none of the studies finds convincing evidence of adverse effects, cries will be raised that the studies were incompetently done at best and coverups at worst. More studies will be suggested and demanded. It could go on for a long time, but I think that the decision that has already been made—that dioxin has not caused life-threatening human diseases—will defuse the requests for more studies, rendering them superfluous.

Whereas courts can be satisfied that no harm has been done

if no harm can be demonstrated, the EPA is charged with protecting us from small risks. 2,4,5-T may no longer be manufactured, but dioxin still remains in the environment. The action in the years to come will be in the regulatory arena; the EPA is moving ahead with a strategy to identify sites of dioxin contamination in the environment. As each site is found, the EPA will have to act.

The word "dioxin" has a far broader meaning than the one chemical that this book has discussed. The dioxin that I have focused on is *only one of 75 chlorinated dioxins*, but it, the chemical 2,3,7,8-tetrachlorodibenzo-*p*-dioxin, is the most toxic dioxin of them all. Further broadening the scope of our concern are two groups of closely related chemicals called *furans* and *polychlorinated biphenyls (PCBs)*. These chemicals share common sizes and shapes with the dioxins and cause the same kinds of toxic effects in laboratory animals. As a general rule, dioxins are more toxic than furans, and furans are more toxic than PCBs. Furan differs from dioxin only in that it contains one less oxygen. Burning PCBs produces dioxins and furans, and because of that, the EPA has imposed strict regulations on electrical equipment containing PCBs, which might ignite.[16]

Testing and studying all 75 chlorinated dioxins and 135 chlorinated furans with the intensity focused on the most toxic dioxin would tie up all the world's toxicologists and epidemiologists for years to come. Rather, researchers have already carried out a few quick tests on some of the other dioxins and furans. Comparison of their results with results obtained with dioxin in the same tests has produced a relative ranking of toxicities.

The comparisons have important ramifications for municipal waste incinerators. The other dioxins and the furans, though not so toxic as dioxin, are more concentrated in fires, making them, according to some analyses, comparable risks. Using the toxicities that have been estimated for these chemicals, the total cancer risk from municipal incinerators might be six times the risk estimated for dioxin alone.[17] But this estimate depends on many assumptions and few data, and it has already been challenged. In particular, if the cancer risk from dioxin is exaggerated, all the other risks are exaggerated. The EPA notes the weak underpinnings for this estimate, but contends that some method is necessary to provide a tool for estimating risks. In contrast, Germany has decided to ignore the possible health effects of other dioxins and furans. Basing its risk estimate only on dioxin, Germany has concluded that municipal waste emissions do not pose a health risk.[18]

The fact that other dioxins as well as furans are more common and/or more readily accumulated by humans is illustrated by some results from Sweden. Seven people who had an average of 3 parts per trillion of dioxin in their fat had concentrations of other dioxins and furans as much as 100 times higher.[19]

Even though we are apparently exposed to more of the other dioxins and to more of the furans, they will not push dioxin out of the news. Its reputation as the most toxic chemical manufactured will keep it in the public eye, with the others vying for attention.

CHAPTER 16

THE PRESENT AND THE FUTURE

Dow announced its decision to stop manufacturing the herbicide 2,4,5-T in October 1983. As the last domestic manufacturer of 2,4,5-T, Dow maintains that the herbicide has not harmed humans. Nevertheless, the management of Dow decided to stop production because of the widespread publicity about the herbicide's health risks, the resultant decreasing sales, and the costs of carrying the legal and scientific fight against the suspension by the Environment Protection Agency (EPA) of the use of 2,4,5-T. The EPA's efforts to regulate the herbicide had begun in 1972, were interrupted in 1974, and reinitiated in 1978. Dow ceased its production more than 10 years after the EPA first tried to regulate it.

Dow's announcement that it was stopping the manufacture and the fight against the EPA was, ironically, made public on the first day of a symposium at Rockefeller University on the "Public Health Risks of the Dioxins." In summarizing the presentations at that meeting, the chairman, William Lowrance, wrote:

> Without question, the dioxins are extraordinarily toxic to rodents and other lower animal species, as is clear from many of the papers in this symposium.
>
> However, despite passionate concern on the part of many possibly exposed individuals, and despite extensive scientific investigation, it is not obvious that the compounds are so toxic to humans. . . . Epidemiologic follow-

ups have not yet convincingly revealed any increased or
unusual pattern of mortality from human exposure. . . .

Thus the dioxins pose a classic public health dilemma:
they are extremely toxic to test animals, but are not clearly
so toxic to humans. Human experience is accumulating
only slowly. Moreover, most of the human exposures appear to have been very small, and have been incurred under circumstances, such as accidents, sporadic spraying,
and war conditions, that make scientific analysis of the exposures and effects very difficult.[1]

No papers published since the Rockefeller University symposium have gone against the tide of data and opinion that
environmental exposures to dioxin have not caused demonstrable human harm. Rather, the investigations of Ranch Hands
have buttressed the conclusion that neither environmentally exposed nor Agent-Orange-exposed people have been harmed.
As mentioned earlier, from the standpoint of regulatory processes, failure to demonstrate harm makes little difference. Congress established the EPA to protect us from environmental
risks, and identifying risks does not require demonstrating
harm. In a similar protective vein, Congress added the Delaney
Clause to the Food, Drug, and Cosmetic Act in 1958, requiring
the Food and Drug Administration (FDA) to remove additives
from food if the additives caused cancer in laboratory animals.
To protect us from risks, Federal agencies can rely on animal
evidence for risk; they do not have to wait for demonstrated
human harm to take action.

The EPA's eventual success in stopping manufacture of
2,4,5-T has reduced dioxin exposures. No workers are now at
risk from explosions or leaks in trichlorophenol or 2,4,5-T
plants; herbicide sprayers, farmers, and forestrymen do not
work with 2,4,5-T, and bystanders cannot be exposed directly
from spray drift or indirectly from spray reaching their food or
water. Pockets of dioxin remain in chemical disposal dumps,
around plants that formerly produced trichlorophenol or 2,4,
5-T, and, in much, much lower concentrations, where 2,4,5-T
was sprayed in the environment. In addition to the sources of
"old" dioxin, "new" dioxin is coming from fires of various

kinds. This source will never equal the rate of dioxin produced as a by-produce of trichlorophenol production, but it will add to the environmental burden.

By now, much of the dioxin in dumps and the general environment is firmly attached to particles of soil. Although binding between dioxin and soil is so tight that little of the chemical will leach into water supplies, there is concern about low levels of dioxin in water. Each adult drinks about two liters (about two quarts) of water daily. Moreover, people are directly exposed to dioxin in the soil through dust blown onto their skin, some fraction of which is absorbed through the skin. Dioxin-laced dust can also be inhaled or even ingested. Children are at greater risk here, for many enjoy playing in dirt and tend to put their hands and fingers in their mouths.

Indirectly, we may be exposed to dioxin from soil by eating animals that have ingested dioxin-laced soil. The FDA has estimated that bottom-living fish, such as carp and catfish, are more likely to carry dioxin because their feeding habits include sucking up soil particles.[2] Furthermore, fish that live in water containing dioxin concentrate it in their tissues.[3] When people eat the fish, they will be exposed to the dioxin as well. In terms of livestock, swine might be most contaminated because they routinely ingest soil with their food.[4]

No Federal agency regulates the levels of dioxin in soil, fish, or water, but the Centers for Disease Control (CDC),[5] FDA,[6] and EPA[7] have calculated "virtually safe doses" for dioxin in these materials. In 1981, the FDA advised the Great Lake states that no one should eat fish that contained dioxin at levels greater than 50 *parts per trillion (ppt)*, no one should eat fish that contained dioxin at 25–50 ppt more than twice a month, and fish with less than 25 ppt could be eaten without restriction. Although the FDA's suggestions are not binding, they were prepared at the request of the Great Lakes states that wanted advice about what levels were acceptable, and because of that, the FDA assumes that the states will test fish for dioxin. A state can test a sampling of fish from each major fishing area and, depending on the results, allow or not allow fish from areas to be sold. The FDA-recommended level has a practical side; at a cost of $1000 per sample, analytical chemistry can reliably detect dioxin at levels no lower than about 10 ppt in fish. Therefore, 25 ppt is a level that can be measured. Furthermore, since only some fish from each fishery have to be sampled, the costs of sampling would seem manageable.

Concentrations of dioxin as high as 300 *parts per billion (ppb)* were found in soil under roadways in Times Beach, Missouri, where wastes from trichlorophenol plants were sprayed. Although concentrations were much lower in areas adjacent to people's homes, a decision had to be made about a safe level. The CDC calculated a virtually safe dose for people who lived on contaminated soil their entire lives, were exposed as children when playing in the dirt, and ate some food grown on the contaminated soil. According to the CDC's calculation, soil contaminated at 1 ppb might increase people's risk of cancer by one in a million. Since about 20% of Americans die of cancer, each of us has about a 20% chance of dying of it. If we add a one-in-a-million additional risk to this risk, the risk increases to 20.0001%. In terms of populations, if a million people were exposed to 1 ppb, no more than one of them would be expected to develop cancer from that exposure. Of course, if environmental concentrations of dioxin did cause one additional cancer in a million people, the increase would be undetectable.

I have heard that the CDC actually settled on the 1 ppb level for the practical reason that it was the lowest level that could be reliably detected in dirt. I have also been told that the level was selected because it would justify the Federal government's buying out of Times Beach. At the time of the buyout, the EPA was under spirited attack for inattention to the environment—Ann Burford was under Congressional pressure to resign and Rita Lavelle was facing contempt of Congress charges. It has been suggested that the action at Times Beach was partly motivated by a desire to show that the EPA was doing something. Whether or not either or both of these rumors is correct, the official justification for the decision was a CDC risk assessment that concluded that 1 ppb was a level of concern and concentrations less than that were virtually safe doses.

The CDC, the agency that calculated the virtually safe limit at Times Beach, is part of the Department of Health and Human Services. It is separate from the EPA, which is a free-standing agency, not part of any department. The division of responsibility between them at Times Beach will probably become a permanent operating procedure, with the CDC doing the health risk assessment around waste sites, such as Times Beach, and the EPA taking action to protect people from the risk.

The EPA's virtually safe limit for dioxin in water is virtually impossible to understand because it is so infinitesimal; it is 13 parts per quintillion, or 13 parts of dioxin in 1,000,000,000,000,-000,000 parts of water. This quantity is so small that it cannot be measured, which is a source of some embarrassment; how can the EPA protect us from a risk that cannot be measured? In any case, the lowest concentration of dioxin that can be detected in water today, in the parts-per-quadrillion range, is about 100 times greater than the virtually safe limit.

All these infinitesimal quantities strain the imagination. If there were one blue-eyed person in China, he or she would be one part per billion in that population. I have no illustration of one part per trillion or per quadrillion, but John Moore,[8] assistant administrator of the EPA, has suggested an illustration of one part per quintillion. If McDonald's continues making hamburgers at its current rate, it will take 1 billion years for it to make one quintillion burgers. Locating one particular burger in that immense pile would be equivalent to finding one part of dioxin in one quintillion parts of water.

The amounts of dioxin that would be taken up by a person exposed to the three virtually safe doses—computed by FDA for fish, by CDC for soil, and EPA for water—are different, even though all the estimates are based on the carcinogenicity of dioxin in rats as determined by Dow scientists[9] and the same general calculations.[10] Consumption of water contaminated at the EPA's virtually safe limit would result in ingesting 0.42 picogram of dioxin (a picogram is $\frac{1}{1},000,000,000,000$ gram); at the FDA's limit for fish, the amount would be about 30 times greater, 13 picograms, and at the CDC's limit for soil, still higher, 45 picograms.

Many assumptions are included in the calculations that produced the estimates of virtually safe doses. In particular, all are based on the occurrence of cancer in rats exposed to dioxin. There is no evidence from humans to support these estimates, nor is there any direct evidence to say that they are incorrect, although they almost certainly exaggerate risk. The exaggeration is built into the computations to provide a margin of safety.

Humans concentrate dioxin in their fat, and a sample of about two teaspoons of human fat, which can be obtained surgically or with a large hypodermic needle and syringe, can be analyzed for dioxin at a cost of about $1000. Knowing how much dioxin is present in humans, scientists can calculate how much dioxin has to be ingested or absorbed to account for that amount. Given that concentrations of dioxin in the fat of Americans and Canadians average about 5 or 10 parts per trillion,[11] the daily intake of dioxin for a person with 5 parts per trillion is somewhere between 95 and 1160 picograms per day,[12] depending on the rate at which dioxin is eliminated from the body. Even 95 picograms is greater than CDC's virtually safe limit for soil which few of us are exposed to.

Finding that an average body burden of dioxin is 5–10 ppt presents a singular difficult question. Where does it come from? First of all, the computation that relates intake to concentrations in body fat may be incorrect. If this is the case, lower exposure levels might be sufficient to produce 5–10 ppt. Although the formula[13] was published in 1976, and has been used since, it is based on studies in animals, and it is possible that it does not accurately depict the relationship between human intake and accumulation. One posssible inaccuracy is that the time necessary for excretion may be longer than estimated in the formula, and there is some evidence for that. Another possible explanation is that the people with 10 ppt dioxin in their fat were exposed to concentrations of dioxin much above the virtually safe levels during the years of heavy 2,4,5-T use. While that seems unlikely, there are no measurements of past exposures.

It is almost certain, if the calculation is correct, that current concentrations of dioxin in soil, water, and fish cannot account for the body burden of dioxin. Soil concentrations above 1 ppb have been found only around chemical plants that formerly made trichlorophenol and 2,4,5-T, near waste disposal sites, and in former chemical storage areas. It is extremely unlikely that anyone who lives at any distance from these sites is exposed to much dioxin from soil. If concentrations of dioxin in fish and water were much higher than the virtually safe doses, drinking water and eating fish could account for the 10 ppt body burden. However, analytical chemists have found that only a fraction of the fish from the Great Lakes and their tributaries ever had concentrations above 25 ppt,[14] the virtually safe limit. Furthermore, according to the FDA, concentrations of dioxin in Great Lakes fish are decreasing, and dioxin is not detected in fish taken from other waters in the United States.[15] Given that fish concentrate dioxin by a factor of 5000, dioxin concentrations in water are much lower than in fish. Even if exposures from water were 100 or 1000 times higher than the EPA's virtually safe level for water, these tiny concentrations would make little contribution to the amount of dioxin ingested.

Finally, there may be other sources of dioxin. Exposures to fire-produced airborne dioxin can contribute some amount to body burden, and they may make a significant contribution to the body burden. Another possible source of exposure is foodstuffs other than fish. Dioxin might be present in beef and pork from animals feeding on contaminated soil or plants, and even plants might take it up. Measurements, however, have only infrequently detected dioxin even in beef that as cattle had grazed on 2,4,5-T-sprayed rangeland. In plants, such as beans and corn, experiments have demonstrated that they take up very little if any dioxin from the soil.[16] Therefore, the possibility of people eating significant amounts of dioxin from sources other than fish is small. With less dioxin being introduced into the environment, the level of dioxin should drop.

There is no clear answer to the question of where the dioxin in human fat comes from. Considering this problem is made more difficult because some people have no detectable body burden of dioxin. Of 13 Swedes classified as occupationally exposed to dioxin in herbicides, 5 had no detectable dioxin in their fat. Furthermore, the average amounts of dioxin found in the fat of Swedes classified as exposed were the same as the amounts found in those classified as occupationally unexposed.[17] While it could be that the classifications are incorrect, we are left with the thorny observation that many, but not all, people have a body burden of dioxin.

What does a body burden of 5 or 10 ppt mean? Some people argue that any level of dioxin might cause cancer and that a person with 5 or 10 ppt is at increased risk. However, we have some data about dioxin concentrations in rats exposed to enough dioxin to cause cancer, and the concentrations are about 8000 ppt, 800 times higher than 10 ppt. In rats exposed to a dose 10-fold lower—which caused no excess cancers in 100 tested rats—the concentration in fat was 1700 ppt. (Dioxin concentrations were even higher in rat livers: 24,000 ppt at the dose that caused liver cancer and 5100 ppt at the lower dose.) Clearly, the human levels are well below those associated with cancer in rats.

Nevertheless, a 10 ppt body burden can be equated with a cancer risk in humans. According to the formula that relates ingested dioxin to body burden, a person would have to take in 100–2000 times the EPA's virtually safe dose to accumulate 10 ppt. Now, if the virtually safe dose, which, it must be remembered, is based on animal data, actually causes one additional cancer in a population of one million people, a dose of 200 or 2000 times higher would be expected to cause 200 or 2000 cancers in a million people. Neither frequency would be detected against the background of 250,000 or more cancers that would be the usual number in a million Americans, unless it caused a relatively rare cancer that would stand out against the background. Therefore, it is possible that a body burden of 10 ppt dioxin is associated with increased cancer risk. It is also possible that such a burden has no effect whatsoever.

Three things are important to remember about measured body burdens in connection with dioxin. There seems to be no association between the amounts of dioxin in humans and whether or not they have a history of exposure to herbicides. No correlation has been found between human body burdens of dioxin and illness. And whatever the body burdens are now, they can be expected to decrease because of the discontinuation of 2,4,5-T production.

Paradoxically, as the level of dioxin in fish, water, and soil decreases, the reports of discoveries of dioxin will probably increase. With improvements in analytical chemistry, more samples will be found to contain dioxin. When we could detect dioxin only at concentrations of one part per million or more, materials containing 0.1 part per million were classified as having nondetectable dioxin; now that we can measure concentrations about a billion times more dilute, fewer samples fall into the nondetectable classification. As I mentioned before, on the basis of animal studies, the EPA estimates a one-in-a-million extra risk of cancer at concentrations of dioxin in water that are about 100 times below the current detection limit. Some day, we will be able to detect that smaller amount. What will we do in response? Will we say that we have gone too far in chasing after tiny risks and reconsider our risk estimates to account for the fact that much higher exposure levels have caused no detectable harm in humans? Or will we declare that the risk must be addressed and begin building water treatment plants to reduce dioxin to still lower concentrations? I think that the country will follow some variant of the former course, having grown weary of reducing risks projected from animal studies and not having detected any serious harm in humans.

More identifications will also result from a systematic look for dioxin in the environment. Responding to public and congressional concern about exposures, the EPA, in late 1983, published *Dioxin Strategy*[18], which detailed plans to pinpoint sources of dioxin exposures. The EPA listed potential sites of exposure in seven tiers or categories from the greatest threats to the least—the first tier being former production sites, tiers two through six being places in which herbicides were mixed or used or disposed of as well as combustion sites, and tier seven being places in which people live and in which dioxin would be unexpected.

Dioxin is not everywhere. Not even all sites in which trichlorophenol and herbicides were manufactured, mixed, used, and disposed of are contaminated.[19] Most important to the general population, the maximum contamination found in soil from areas in which there is no history of commercial activities involving dioxin has been less than ¹⁄₁₀₀th of the one-part-per-billion level in soil that CDC established as a level of concern.

The EPA has also sampled dioxin in fish throughout the country. Only 1 fish, taken in Maine, of all places, exceeded the FDA's 25 ppt level of concern; 5 more were over 10 ppt, and the remaining 39 with any detectable dioxin were under 10 ppt. The remaining 155 of 200 sampled fish contained no detectable dioxin. All the positive samples from the Great Lakes and tributaries were less than 25 ppt, reinforcing the FDA's conclusion that dioxin levels are decreasing in fish from that area. With all the safety factors built into the calculations of the CDC's and FDA's levels of concern, the scattered and low-level detections of dioxin are reassuring that the general public is at little risk of exposure to high levels of dioxin.

Fire-generated dioxin is taking on more significance. Mountains of municipal, commercial, and industrial waste are being burned. More will be burned, because waste incineration offers an alternative to dumping waste into the ground, which endangers surface and groundwater supplies. As more waste fires burn and are planned, even in the most sophisticated furnaces, concern about dioxin production is bound to rise.

New York City's garbage problems are familiar to everyone who has a television set. During the city's garbage strikes, the sight of heaps of bursting bags and overstuffed garbage cans teetering on the curbs reinforces for many Americans that New York City is a place only to visit. After trying to imagine and consider terribly tiny quantities like picograms, trying to imagine New York's garbage problem is an exercise in the opposite direction. Each day the city generates 28,000 tons (that is, 56 million pounds) of garbage. About 5000 tons, largely commercial waste, are collected by private refuse companies and hauled out of the city for disposal or burning. The remaining 23,000 tons are collected by the city's Sanitation Department and deposited in two large landfills. The landfills are a delight to the gulls that scavenge on the south shore of Long Island. But these landfills are beginning to fill up and will have to be closed in a few years. Unfortunately, garbage will not stop coming simply because there is no place to dump it.

In addition to decreasing the bulk of wastes, burning waste generates heat, which can be used to produce steam that, in turn, can be sold to electrical generating companies. With this in mind, New York City has planned a number of "resource recovery" plants. Their attraction is the selling of steam to recapture part of the capital and operating costs of the plants. Still, the presence of dioxin in the plant's emissions is a thorn in an otherwise rosy picture.

New York City's Board of Estimates approved the building of the first of five resource recovery plants at the end of 1984. The approval followed a spirited objection to the plant that included an estimate that the plant would increase lung cancer rates by 8%.[20] When made aware of the possible dioxin risk, the Board of Estimates requested the Department of Sanitation to review the literature about dioxin from municipal incinerators and the cancer risk from dioxin. The department placed a contract with an engineering firm to investigate the risks. As part of its contract, the engineering firm assembled a panel of nine experts in engineering, public health, and risk assessment to review the report it produced.[21] The report, released in the fall of 1984, estimated a total of between less than one and six extra cancers per million people who were continually exposed to the maximum level of emissions for 70 years. Again, the cancer estimate is based on cancer rates determined in rodents exposed to dioxin and calculated by standard methods. The review panel approved the report, and the report was well received by the Board of Estimates, according to the Director of Public Policy of the Sanitation Department. In his opinion, inclusion of the review by independent experts convinced the board that whatever risks exist are acceptable.

The first incinerator will be installed at the Brooklyn Navy Yard after a citizens' panel from Brooklyn reviewed and generally approved the plans for the facility. The Sanitation Department wisely provided funds to the panel so it could hire its own experts.[22] This act, I think, was important to public acceptance of the plans. Without access to experts, the public often finds itself at a great disadvantage in technical discussions. Given its own experts, the public knows that its opinions will be informed and counted.

The Board of Estimates voted (6 to 5) on August 15, 1985, to allow the Department of Sanitation to begin writing contracts for construction of the plant that will eventually burn 3000 tons of garbage daily. Additionally, plans are going ahead for four more resource recovery facilities, one in each of the other boroughs. A planned total of eight facilities, each with a 3000-ton daily capacity, will be sufficient to dispose of all the city's garbage.

Temperatures of about 1600°F are necessary to keep dioxin emissions in the range that produced the acceptable estimate of fewer than six extra cancers per million people. No matter how well designed the furnace, care in maintenance and operation is necessary to carry this out successfully. To guarantee that these conditions are met, the plant will require a permit from the State Department of Environmental Conservation. If the emissions limit is exceeded, the plant will be closed down.[23]

It is still possible that the construction of the incinerators will slow or stop because of dioxin or some other problem. However, the diligence of the Sanitation Department in assembling technical information and in cooperating with citizens to provide them with independent sources of expertise has apparently paved the way for construction. I think that the openness of the process, involving citizens and especially providing them with access to experts of their choosing, is a critical feature to the progress of this program in New York City. Nevertheless, not everyone in New York accepted the decision of the Board of Estimates, and some Brooklyn citizens planned to go to court to stop construction.

The New York City effort may become an important model for many other cities. If it works and demonstrates that incineration is not necessarily accompanied by signficant dioxin emissions, such facilities will probably be built elsewhere. In addition, should the public and experts ever decide that the risk of dioxin is exaggerated, cities will be able to build incinerators to less stringent standards, at less cost, and without the level of controversy with which the New York City proposal was met.

Before turning from incineration, it is worth mentioning again that it is a good, if expensive, method to dispose of dioxin-contaminated material. In July 1985, the EPA announced that its mobile incinerator can burn a ton of solid and liquid waste an hour and destroy 99.9999% of the dioxin it contains. Dioxin destruction by this method costs between $200 and $1200 a ton of contaminated material. Neither the ash left after burning nor the gases emitted from the incinerator are hazardous. The EPA hopes that private industry will improve on the incinerator and produce more efficient models.[24]

One of the most widely used insulators in electrical equipment, commonly known as PCBs (polychlorinated biphenyls), generates dioxin when burned. Although PCBs are no longer manufactured in this country, many electrical transformers containing PCBs remain in service. In at least three buildings, soot generated by fires in basement transformers was sucked up by the air-conditioning system and blown throughout the building. The best-known incident was the February 5, 1981, fire in a state office building in Binghamton, New York. The soot, which spread throughout 18 floors, contained up to 3 parts per million dioxin,[25] which is about one and a half times the average concentration of dioxin in Agent Orange.

The building remained closed for more than 4 years while the soot was removed, much of the interior of the building was replaced, and all surfaces with which humans might come in contact were removed or covered. In the spring of 1985, scientists measured dioxin levels in the air of the building, and an advisory panel reviewed the results in mid-August 1985. Although very low concentrations of dioxin remained, the decision was made to reopen the building because they were judged not to present a significant risk.

The PCB fires have added a new dimension to hazards in the workplace. In the past, almost all workers in factories where there was potential exposure to dioxin were men. Today, many workers in office buildings are women. No convincing evidence exists that environmental exposures to dioxin have caused miscarriages or other reproductive health effects. However, the possibility that PCB fires cause levels of dioxin higher than those from spraying has led to concern about effects on women's reproduction. I doubt that any woman will be allowed in the buildings before the levels of dioxin are reduced to a level that experts agree will not cause harm, but I think that the renewed attention to reproductive health is a harbinger of changing emphasis on dioxin's health effects—away from cancer and toward other effects.

No convincing evidence links exposure to dioxin with cancer. Vietnam veterans were unable to substantiate or sustain the claims that Agent Orange caused their cancers. And, as noted repeatedly, consideration of the calculated risk of cancer along with exposure levels makes it unlikely that an association could be demonstrated even if one exists. Acceptance of these conclusions leads one to question why calls for additional studies of exposed people continue to be heard. The usual answer is two-sided: First, additional studies might identify so-far unknown associations between dioxin and cancer; second, if no associations are found, the results will reassure the study subjects and other exposed people. In response, I would say that if effects are there and if they are detectable in any study of humans, especially in men, they would surely have been seen in already-completed studies, or they will be seen in ongoing studies. And although finding no effects might provide reassurance, this could be done more quickly and less expensively by publicizing the results of studies already done.

Another answer to the question of why do more studies often begins, "We have focused too much on men and cancer, ignoring other people and other effects." In particular, there is a shift to concern about women and children and their health. Although we can extrapolate from high-level industrial exposures for males to say that we expect no effects in men from environmental exposures, there are few instances of industrial exposure of women or children.

The biology of women and children differs from that of men; also, the emotional impact of their being at risk may differ. While there may be differences between men and women in susceptibility to disease, the striking difference is the vulnerability of the fetus carried by the pregnant woman. Our earliest information about dioxin toxicity showed its causing fetal poisoning and death in several species of laboratory animals and cleft palates in mice. This information coupled with perceptions of the high risks that pregnant women already encounter leads to questions about the effect of environmental, industrial, or office building exposures on reproductive health.

On the basis of animal studies, virtually safe doses have been established for fetotoxicity in humans. Under the most stringent calculations, these virtually safe doses are somewhat higher than the virtually safe dose for cancer. Therefore, as long as the same limits are observed for exposures that protect against cancer, there will likely be no fetotoxicity. The rub is that while we have numerous studies about human cancer, we have very few about reproductive health effects. With so few, the suggestion that we should do studies to see whether there might be unpredicted human effects seems a reasonable one.

None of the claims about miscarriages and 2,4,5-T spraying has held up when subjected to close scrutiny. Furthermore, these sprayings no longer continue in the United States, so there will be no more of these episodes. But there will be possible exposures from soil and water and fish in some parts of the country, and possibly in buildings after PCB fires. The relatively high exposure level of pregnant women at Seveso is judged not to have increased the number of spontaneous abortions, but that one-time very high exposure is not exactly analogous to continual exposures at lower levels. Hence, our facts about miscarriages and dioxin are sketchy at best.

Moreover, the occurrence of miscarriages is difficult to study. The researchers who carried out the elaborate, expensive, and careful study of survivors of the bombings of Hiroshima and Nagasaki and their children were forced to abandon their attempts to count spontaneous abortions. The difficulties of classifying and recording were overwhelming. Depending on people's recall or even medical records about spontaneous abortion, as we emphasized before, has proved unsatisfactory time after time. A woman who wanted to be pregnant may remember a late period as a miscarriage; a woman who did not want to be pregnant may not remember the event at all. Medical records can help but not without special attention and preparation. Record-keeping differs from area to area, hospital to hospital, doctor to doctor. Still, with all the anticipated difficulties, new studies of the possible dioxin–spontaneous abortion link will probably be undertaken. No number of calculations that show that the study is likely to find nothing will convince all concerned not to go ahead. In particular, I expect that there will be a lot of attention given to spontaneous abortions in areas around waste dumps, many of which contain some amount of dioxin.

A second area of new emphasis will be neurological disease. The incapacitating aches and pains and irritability of workers who have been highly exposed demonstrate that dioxin can affect the nervous system. Do chronic exposures at lower levels have the same consequences? On one plane, this is an open question. We know little in general about neurotoxins—poisons that especially harm the nervous system—and even less about their possible effects at low exposure levels. About dioxin in particular, we have conflicting results about nonreparable nerve damage. One Nitro worker's clinically measured neurological damage persisted from the 1949 accident at least through the time he was examined as part of a study in 1979. Although scientists do not know whether dioxin caused the problems, since he may have been exposed to other chemicals, he was one of the workers most affected by dioxin. As in the case of spontaneous abortions, effects on the nervous system are difficult to study. Furthermore, aches and pains are real, whether they can be measured or not. They can also have a variety of causes or, as we all know, no cause that we can identify. A sore arm after playing catch on the first warm day of spring or an aching back the day after helping someone move is easily explainable. But sometimes, an arm or leg or jaw or back just hurts and even depression and gloom sometime seem to come from nowhere.

It is possible to gather information about aches and pains and emotional states by questioning people in a rigorously controlled setting. However, if I knew I had been exposed to dioxin and that I might receive compensation for it or some assistance in removing a waste site from the neighborhood in which my kids were growing up, I would do a very serious inventory of my aches, pains, and feelings. Such human foibles complicate the process of health surveys.

I think that environmental exposure to dioxin is unlikely to have caused damage to the nervous system, but the possibility remains open. I firmly disagree that we will learn much about the possible effects of dioxin on the nervous system by studying people who may have been environmentally exposed. The levels are too low. A study by the National Institute for Occupational Safety and Health of workers who were exposed to dioxin is much more likely to provide us with some useful information. Only if effects were found in such a group, would I expect a study of environmental exposures to teach us anything.

Given a choice, I would prefer that no one be exposed to dioxin and that no one have a body burden of dioxin. Many of us have been exposed and many of us have a body burden, which means we may be at some risk of disease. There is no way to wave a magic wand and make dioxin disappear from the environment, but we know it is decreasing, and any risks that poses should be going down as well. At greater expense and with greater effort, we could reduce risks faster, by tightening up on incineration, by scraping up and burning soil, and by other measures. However, in the absence of demonstrated human harm from environmental exposures, not to mention the discontinued manufacturing of the primary source of dioxin, I believe that the amount being spent and the effort being expended are certainly sufficient.

The shift of emphasis from dioxin's causing cancer to its possibly causing spontaneous abortions and neurological damage is symptomatic of the cascade of effects blamed on dioxin and other chemicals in the environment. Little evidence is needed to invoke an association between an exposure and a new disease or problem, but a lot of effort may be required to investigate it. There is a need to investigate real possibilities of harm to protect the public, but there is a point at which such studies become useless. For years, many people accepted that cancer is the disease most to be feared from low-level exposures. Yet no link has been found to substantiate a link between dioxin and cancer. Since it has not, I expect that no other effects will be found either. Scientists found none at Seveso, and the American Medical Association concluded that the only health problem definitely associated with dioxin is chloracne and that it has come only from high occupational exposures.[26]

Even in the absence of any demonstrated serious harm, people who are worried about dioxin's risks want more epidemiological studies to search for damage to humans. Most of the studies done to date have been "fishing expeditions" that look for any effect whatsoever. In 1985, both the congressional Office of Technology Assessment and the White House Agent Orange Working Group declared that the time was past for fishing expeditions. Those studies had failed to find any effects and to do more would be wasteful. Focused studies, such as those to investigate the possible association between dioxin and soft tissue sarcomas or between dioxin and nervous system damage in highly exposed workers, or studies about possible mechanisms of disease causation, may be considered, but studies simply to gather general data will not be.

Despite all that has been learned, the clamor that surrounds the topic of dioxin invites the question of what should be done differently and better in identifying, measuring, and managing environmental risks. In my mind, the answers are general, ranging far beyond issues of toxic chemicals, but they are rooted in the specific. The identification and quantification of health hazards is accomplished by scientists, and scientists often disagree. With more data and more discussion, scientists reach a consensus or, at least, edge toward it with "great uncertainty" and by using many variations of the phrase "on the other hand." There are outlyers who remain apart from the consensus. Some outlyers have been right in the past; some of the most famous scientists are those who broke with the middle and staked out new ground. But more generally, outlyers are an extreme, eventually cast aside as the middle opinions grow more robust and certain. *The position of the majority of scientists who have examined the human health effects of dioxin is that little or no harm has been done.*[27]

Still, outlyers, who see dioxin as a cause of life-threatening human disease, can go to the public with the message, "I know what causes your afflictions. You have a reason for your fears. Someone is to blame. Together we will identify the perpetrator and see that this never happens again." A powerful message. Identifying causes is often the first step in reducing human misery. The message is understandably more attractive if the cause does not reside in a person's own biology and is outside his own responsibility. In addition to the appeal of the message, the very role of outlyer has its own charm, seen and often self-portrayed as a brave crusader against monolithic conventional wisdom.

These are bad times for conventional wisdom, especially when it supports the position of the government or corporate America, which have given us good reason to distrust them. When scientists' work supports industry's or government's position, the distrust can extend to encompass the scientists and their work as well. So long as that happens, Congress and the regulatory agencies will at least consider public policy about chemical hazards and other environmental risks that run along tracks near the outlyers' positions. There is a certain good in this state of affairs; risks will be reduced. It is not all good, however, because of inefficiencies when more is spent than is necessary. Neither is it good if it frightens people unnecessarily or if it raises their hopes too high about what will be accomplished by reducing exposures to the risk. Dioxin has caused little demonstrable harm, and environmental exposures may have caused no health effects. Because there was little or no harm, the amount of money and effort spent on controlling dioxin may be completely out of line with any improvement in human health. I do not subscribe to the position that had we spent less effort on dioxin we would have spent more on other hazards and be farther along in cleaning up the environment. Dioxin has a special place. Had we not put so much effort into it, we would more likely have done pretty much what we did about other things. It did not, I think, detract from other efforts; it added to them.

Restoring respect for authority on the basis of scientific fact and opinion is difficult when disrespect for authority is the generic condition of the American public. However, the country's decision-making processes have incorporated the scientific consensus in reaching some conclusions about dioxin.

The CDC's study of birth defects among children of Vietnam veterans, which found no convincing evidence of effects, was instrumental in assuaging congressional concern about birth defects and influenced the judge's decision in the Agent Orange lawsuit. That study was well done, extensively reviewed by government and nongovernment scientists, and published in the *Journal of the American Medical Association*. All the care and notice promoted its acceptance. The Air Force's study of men who sprayed Agent Orange has not had so pronounced an impact because the exposure of those men was different from that of most veterans. However, scientists have extensively reviewed it and have generally accepted its conclusions. Going the extra mile to make facts and opinions open to scrutiny seems to be the method by which existing scientific research can best be used to convince the public that environmental exposures to dioxin, despite whatever risks they may harbor, have not caused human harm.

In contrast to dioxin, many decisions about environmental risks are made with little public attention and less controversy. In my mind, at least, the level of controversy may be more related to having someone or some organization to blame for the risk than to the level of risk. For instance, the biggest looming environmental problem is probably radon gas that escapes from the earth and enters people's basements in some parts of the country. Sometimes levels of radioactivity in such homes is greater than the maximal occupational limit. On the basis of what is known about radon causing human cancer and the radioactivity in those homes, scientists estimate that these exposures may cause 10,000[28] to 20,000[29] deaths annually. These very large numbers may attract the public's attention, but there will be no court cases or anyone to blame for the exposures. Without health risk being coupled with legal proceedings and accusations of wrongdoing, radon will not achieve the high visibility of dioxin.

Our society is exposed to invisible, undetectable chemicals and afflicted with diseases. The linking of exposures to "new" and incompletely characterized chemicals with diseases that have obscure origins seems a reasonable assumption. However, the saga of dioxin shows that simply linking exposure and a group of diseases may provoke unnecessary and unrealistic alarm and fear. After a decade and a half of studies and debates, harm from environmental exposure to dioxin has been assessed as nondetectable. Although concern about risk remains, exposures have been reduced, so that the level of risk has decreased. The consensus among most scientists—that harm has been limited to highly exposed industrial populations and that none has been shown from environmental exposures—may often be ignored, and the old claims about harm will be brought up again and gain. But I am confident that the information gathered by science will eventually prevail. We are putting the dioxin problem behind us.

CALCULATION OF THE AMOUNT OF DIOXIN EXPOSURE OF A PERSON STANDING UNDER A RANCH HAND SPRAY MISSION

The numbers in the table below are results of calculating[1] the amount of dioxin that would fall on a man's head and shoulders if he were standing in the open or in a jungle below a Ranch Hand spray mission. Three different estimates were made because neither I nor anyone else knows the concentration of dioxin in Agent Orange. The concentrations of 50, 2, and 0.5 parts per million (ppm) were chosen because 47 ppm was the

Estimated Amounts of Dioxin That Would Fall on a Man from a Ranch Hand Spray Mission

Concentration of dioxin in Agent Orange	Amount of dioxin on a man standing in:	
	The open	The jungle[a]
50 parts per million	32.4 micrograms	1.94 micrograms
2 parts per million	1.3 micrograms	0.08 microgram
0.5 part per million	0.3 microgram	0.02 microgram

[a]About 6% of sprayed Agent Orange reached the jungle floor.

highest concentration ever found in Agent Orange; the average concentration was estimated to be 2 ppm, and the lowest was 0.5 ppm.[2]

We know from studies done in Germany[3] and the United States[4] that the minimum amount of dioxin necessary to cause chloracne is greater than 50 micrograms applied to a small area of the skin. The same amount would probably not cause chloracne if spread over the much larger of the head and shoulders, but even if it did, the amount of dioxin from Ranch Hand sprays is less than that. If the concentration were 50 ppm and the man were standing in the open, the amount of dioxin on him would be 32 micrograms, about half of a dose that is known to be insufficient to cause choracne. Of course, if the concentration were less than 50 ppm, the amount of dioxin on the man would decrease correspondingly. The calculation of the maximal dose as being less than 32 micrograms per man is consistent with the virtual (complete?) absence of reports of chloracne among Vietnam veterans.

According to the Food and Drug Administration[5] (FDA), the virtually safe dose for ingested dioxin is 13 picograms (0.000013 micrograms). The virtually safe dose is a calculated amount: According to the calculation, a person consuming that amount of dioxin daily for 70 years would increase his risk of cancer by one in a million. Stated another way, if a million people were exposed to the virtually safe dose for 70 years, only one (or none) of those people would be expected to develop cancer as a result of that exposure. An added risk of one in a million is acceptable to all regulatory agencies; if the risk is that low, generally they will not act to reduce it still further.

Under the most extreme conditions of a man standing in the open directly under the 50 ppm spray and all the dioxin penetrating into his body, the man would receive about 32.4 micrograms = 32,400,000 picograms or about 2,500,000 times the FDA's virtually safe dose. The other exposures shown in the table are smaller. The most likely amount of exposure, which would be to a man in the jungle under a 2 ppm dioxin spray, would be about 0.08 micrograms = 80,000 picograms or about

6,100 times the virtually safe dose. The lowest exposure, for a man in the jungle under the 0.5 ppm dioxin spray, is just about 1,500 times the FDA's virtually safe dose.

However, having dioxin on a soldier's helmet or hat and uniform is not the same as ingesting it, and the FDA's virtually safe dose is based on ingested dioxin. Stevens[6] has computed that about $\frac{1}{2000}$ of the dioxin in the environment is transferred into the human body. The low efficiency of transfer results from clothing protecting most of the skin from direct contact and from little of the dioxin being on the person's lips where it can be ingested. In the table below, I have assumed that Stevens's computation is correct and that $\frac{1}{2000}$ of the dioxin on the soldier would penetrate his clothing and his skin and enter his body.

Assuming that the efficiency of transfer of dioxin from the environment into a man's body is equal to Stevens's estimate, under the most extreme condition of a soldier in the open under a 50 ppm dioxin spray, the internal dose will be 1,246 times greater than the FDA's virtually safe dose. Under the more realistic conditions of a 2 ppm dioxin spray in the jungle, the internal dose would be 3 times of the virtually safe dose. There is no reason to think that any veteran was exposed to Agent Orange sprays on a daily basis, and, of course, no veteran spent a 70 year lifetime under the sprays.

CDC[8] estimates that the Agent Orange (and dioxin) con-

Comparison of the Amounts of Dioxin Likely To Be Taken up by a Sprayed Soldier's Body with the FDA's Virtually Safe Dose[a]

Dioxin in Agent Orange (ppm)	Dioxin taken up by exposed man[b]			
	Man in open (picograms)	Fraction of FDA's VSD	Man in jungle (picograms)	Fraction of FDA's VSD
50	16,200	1,246	972	75
2	648	50	39	3
0.5	162	12	10	0.7

[a]The virtually safe dose (VSD) is the amount of dioxin that can be ingested daily for 70 years and is calculated to increase the individual's risk of cancer by no more than one chance in a million. The VSD is 13 picograms.
[b]Assuming that the transfer of dioxin from the environment to the inside of the human body is 1/2000, computed by Stevens, 1981.[6]

centration at 0.5 kilometer away from a spray mission would have been no more than 2% of the concentration in the center of the flight path. At 1 kilometer, the concentration would have been no more than 0.03%. Making all the assumptions in the table immediately above, the amount of dioxin taken up by a man 0.5 kilometer from a 50 ppm spray would be 324 picograms. At that distance, only the 50 ppm and 2 ppm sprays in the open would produce doses greater than the FDA's virtually safe dose of 13 picograms. At 1.0 kilometer from a 50 ppm spray, the amount taken up by a man would have been 4.9 picograms.

Dioxin degrades rapidly in sunlight, half of it disappearing in 2 hours. Therefore, any that remained on the surface of vegetation would be rapidly degraded. Dioxin that reached the ground before it degraded would bind to the soil, becoming resistant to degradation. Neither Agent Orange nor dioxin is volatile, and as they reached the ground or landed on plant life, they would no longer be in the man's breathing zone. A veteran could absorb some dioxin from soil that got on his skin or from any that he ingested, but either of those would be a tiny fraction of the amount from a direct spray.

Finally, dioxin could reach water supplies. It is almost insoluble in water, but soldiers who drank contaminated water could have ingested some dioxin. Nevertheless, the dioxin, which is denser than water, would tend to sink to the bottom of any stream or pond and once there bind to soil particles.

At the time Congress ordered that an epidemiological study of veterans be made, its members were not convinced by calculations that exposures were low. There were many claims of veterans being drenched in spray, and certainly there are possibilities that veterans were exposed to higher concentrations through accidents and spills. Six years have passed since Congress ordered the study, and I think that almost everyone who has examined the exposure question is convinced that the men were exposed to amounts of dioxin that are not likely to cause health effects. However, some people remain convinced that dioxin is far more toxic than the FDA estimates and that exposures were much higher. Congress chose to respond to these convictions by carrying out the epidemiological studies of veterans to determine whether their health was affected.

NOTES

CHAPTER 1

1. "Dioxin contamination found at Fort A. P. Hill near site where Boy Scouts camped." *Washington Post*, Nov. 10, 1984. p. B3.
2. *Ibid.*
3. "Scouts plan meeting by dioxin site: Toxic soil found at Fort A. P. Hill." *Washington Post*, November 12, 1984. p. B1.
4. Department of the Army, Office of the Assistant Secretary. Information for Parents of Scouts and Fort A. P. Hill Visitors. Typescript. November 16, 1984.
5. Kimbrough, R. D., H. Falk, P. Stehr, *et al.* Health implications of 2,3,7,8-tetrachlorodibenzo-*p*-dioxin (TCDD) contamination of residential soil. In: *Public Health Risks of the Dioxins*, ed. Lowrance, W. W. (Los Altos, California: William Kaufman, 1984). pp. 121–150; same authors and title. *J. Toxicology Environmental Health* **14**:47–93. 1984.
6. *New York Times.* Nov. 30, 1984. p. B10.

CHAPTER 2

1. Hay, A. *The Chemical Scythe.* (New York: Plenum, 1982), pp. 89–93; G. Reggiana, Interpharco, Ltd., personal communication, July 1985.
2. Interdepartmental Committee on Toxic Chemicals. *Dioxins in Canada: The Federal Approach.* Hull, Quebec: Government of Canada. 1983.
3. Young, A. L., J. A. Calcagni, C. E. Thalken, *et al. The Toxicology, Environmental Fate, and Human Risk of Herbicide Orange and Its Associated Dioxin.* (Washington, D.C.: The Surgeon General, United States Air Force. 1978), p. I-28.
4. Bumb, R., W. Crummet, S. Cutie, *et al.* Trace chemistries of fire: A source of chlorinated dioxins. *Science* **210**:385–390. 1980.
5. Nestrick, T. J., L. L. Lamparski, L. A. Shadoff, *et al.* Methodology and preliminary results for the isomer-specific determination of TCDDs and

higher chlorinated dibenzo-*p*-dioxins in chimney particulates from wood-fueled domestic furnaces located in eastern, central, and western regions of the United States. In: *Human and Environmental Risks of Chlorinated Dioxins and Related Compounds*, eds. Tucker, R. E., A. L. Young, and A. P. Gray (New York: Plenum Press, 1983). pp. 95–112.

6. Wang, D. K. W., D. H. Chiu, P. K. Leung, *et al.* Sampling and analytical methodologies for PCDDs and PCDFs in incinerators and wood burning facilities. In: *Human and Environmental Risks of Chlorinated Dioxins and Related Compounds*, eds. Tucker, R. E., A. L. Young, and A. P. Gray (New York: Plenum Press, 1983). pp. 113–126.

7. Health and Welfare Canada and Environment Canada. Report of the Ministers' Expert Advisory Committee on Dioxins. November, 1983.

8. Dioxin desposits far from the source. *Science News* **126:**297. November 10, 1984.

9. Environmental Protection Agency. Typed report as of 6/26/85.

10. Cohen, B. L., *Before It's Too Late*. (New York: Plenum Press, 1983).

CHAPTER 3

1. Madison, C. "Arms and the men." *National Journal*. 1/12/85. p. 97.

2. Wilcox, F. A. *Waiting for an Army To Die* (New York: Random House, 1983). p. ix.

3. Morison, S. E. *The Oxford History of the American People* (New York: Oxford University Press, 1965). p. 162.

4. Young, A. L., J. A. Calcagni, C. E. Thalken, *et al. The Toxicology, Environmental Fate, and Human Risk of Herbicide Orange and Its Associated Dioxin*. Report OEHL TR-78-92 (Brooks Air Force Base, Texas: USAF Occupational and Environmental Health Laboratory, 1978). p. I-11.

5. Young *et al.* 1978. p. I-18.

6. Young *et al.* 1978. p. I-19.

7. Wilcox, 1983. p. 172.

8. Uhl, M., and T. Ensign. *GI Guinea Pigs* (New York: Wideview Books, 1980). p. 150. Chapter 8 of this book provides additional information about the decisions to eliminate the use of Agent Orange in Vietnam and about some of the personalities involved in them.

9. Meseleson, M. S., A. H. Westing, and J. D. Constable. Background material relevant to presentations at the 1970 annual meeting of the AAAS. Typescript, revised 1-14-71. 48 pp.

10. National Research Council. *The Effects of Herbicides in South Vietnam* (Washington: National Academy of Sciences, 1974).

11. National Research Council, 1974.[10] p. xii.

12. National Research Council, 1974.[10] p. S-12.

13. See Westing, A. H. ed. *Herbicides in War* (Taylor and Francis: London and Philadelphia, 1984).

CHAPTER 4

1. Wilcox, F. A. *Waiting for an Army to Die* (Random House: New York, 1983). Also see Chapter 3.
2. Office of Technology Assessment, United States Congress. *Technologies for Determining Cancer Risks from the Environment* (Washington: Government Printing Office, 1981). Reprinted as *Cancer Risk: Assessing and Reducing the Dangers in Our Society* (Boulder, Colorado: Westview Press, 1982). This report describes and discusses much of the available data about cancer in the United States. It also provides a reasonably complete bibliography for cancer statistics through 1980.
3. Wilcox, 1983.[1] p. 24.
4. The annual incidence of testicular cancer among men 20 through 24, 25 through 29, and 30 through 34 is 6.4, 9.1, and 8.1 cases per 100,000, respectively (Young, J. L., C. L. Percy, A. J. Asire, *et al.* Cancer incidence and mortality in the United States, 1973–1977. *National Cancer Institute Monograph No. 57*. National Cancer Institute: Bethesda, Maryland, 1981. pp. 74–75). The exact age distribution of the men who served in Vietnam is not known, but since the average age of the serviceman there was 19.2 years, 2,000,000 is probably an underestimate of how many were in Vietnam before or during their 20th year. Assuming the number was 2,000,000, we can estimate the number of expected testicular cancers in those Vietnam veterans: As 2,000,000 men age from 20 to 24, we would expect 6.4 cases per 100,000 men per year and since there are 20 times that number of men, there would be 128 cases per year. The annual rate is multiplied by 5 years to produce a total of 640 cases in the five-year span between 20 and 24. The comparable calculation for the 25- to 29- and for the 30- to 34-year-old groups yields answers of 910 and 810. Adding these numbers, we arrive at a total of 2360 expected cases of testicular cancer in veterans who served in Vietnam before their 20th birthday. To this total we would have to add smaller numbers that would be expected in the population of men who were older than 20 when they served there.
5. USAF School of Aerospace Medicine. *Project Ranch Hand II: An Epidemiologic Investigation of Health Effects in Air Force Personnel Following Exposure to Herbicides. Baseline Mortality Study Results* (Brooks Air Force Base, Texas: United States Air Force, 30 June 1983).
6. USAF School of Aerospace Medicine. *Project Ranch Hand II: Mortality Update—1984* (Brooks Air Force Base, Texas: United States Air Force, 1985).
7. *Ibid.*
8. Commonwealth Institute of Health, University of Sydney. *Australian Veterans Health Studies. The Mortality Report. Parts I, II, and III* (Canberra: Australian Government Publishing Service, 1984).
9. See chapter 13.
10. Young, A. L., and H. K. Kang. Status and results of federal epidemiologic studies of populations exposed to TCDD. *Chemosphere*. **14**:779–790. 1985.
11. Greenwald, P., B. Kovasznay, D. N. Collins, *et al.* Sarcomas of soft tissues after Vietnam service. *J. Nat'l Cancer Inst.* **73**:1107–1110. 1984.

12. Kogan, M. D., and R. W. Clapp. Mortality among Vietnam veterans in Massachusetts. Typescript. Massachusetts Office of Commissioner of Veterans Services Agent Orange Program. Jan. 25, 1985.
13. Hajdu, S. I. Classification and pathological diagnosis of soft tissue sarcomas. In: *Public Health Risks of the Dioxins.* ed. W. W. Lowrance (Los Altos, California: William Kaufman, 1984). pp. 173–186.
14. See Chapter 13.
15. *Ibid.*
16. USAF School of Aerospace Medicine. *Project Ranch Hand II: An Epidemiologic Investigation of Health Effects in Air Force Personnel Following Exposure to Herbicides. Baseline Morbidity Study Results* (United States Air Force: Brooks Air Force Base, Texas, 24 February 1984).
17. "The Truth about Agent Orange."*New York Times.* Aug. 13, 1984. p. A22.
18. Interview with Judge Jack Weinstein, Feb. 25, 1985.
19. *Ibid.*
20. "Judge Tentatively Approves Pact on Agent Orange." *New York Times,* Sept. 26, 1984. p. B3.
21. "Agent Orange Payments Plan Limits the Number of Awards." *New York Times,* Feb. 28, 1985. p. B1.
22. United States' memorandum in opposition to defendants' motion for summary judgment based on the government contract defense. Filed in "Agent Orange" Product Liability Litigation. 8/31/84.
23. McCarty, F., President of Vietnam Veterans Agent Orange Victims. Letter to the editor. *New York Times.* May 7, 1985.
24. "The Truth about Agent Orange." *New York Times,* Aug. 13, 1984. p. A22.
25. "Orangemail: Why It Got Paid." *New York Times,* Mar. 8, 1985. p. A34.
26. "Agent Orange Settlement?" *Washington Post,* Mar. 4, 1985. p. A10.
27. "No Bonanza for Lawyers." *Washington Post,* Jan. 15, 1985. p. A10.

CHAPTER 5

1. General Accounting Office. *U.S. Ground Troops in South Vietnam Were in Areas Sprayed with Herbicide Orange* (Government Printing Office: Washington, D.C., November 16, 1979).
2. Phone call to John Hansen, GAO, February 1985.
3. Until November 1985, the members of the Agent Orange Working Group were the Departments of Agriculture, Defense, Health and Human Services, and Labor, the VA, the Environmental Protection Agency, the Office of Management and Budget, and the Office of Science and Technology Policy. The congressional Office of Technology Assessment was the only observer organization, and my colleague Hellen Gelband and I participated in AOWG activities from the beginning. The working group was reduced in size in November 1985.
4. Bricker, J. G. Memorandum for the Chairman, AOWG Science Panel: Proposed Agent Orange troop exposure and non-exposure cohort selection concept paper. Typescript. 4 Dec. 1981.

5. See Chapter 10.
6. See Chapter 13.
7. See Chapter 13.
8. Office of Technology Assessment. Review of Centers for Disease Control *Protocols for Epidemiologic Studies of the Health of Vietnam Veterans.* Typescript. July 1983. pp. 29–30.
9. See Chapter 4.

CHAPTER 6

1. Courtney, K. D., and J. A. Moore. Teratology studies with 2,4,5-trichlorophenoxyacetic acid and 2,3,7,8-tetrachlorodibenzo-*p*-dioxin. *Bull. Environ. Contam. Toxicol.***7**:45–51. 1971.
2. See Chapter 8.
3. Tung, T. T., T. K. Anh, B. Q. Tuyen, *et al.* Clinical effects of massive and continuous utilization of defoliants on civilians. *Vietnamese Studies* **29**:53–81. 1971.
4. Tung, T. T., T. D. Lang, and D. D. Van. The problem of mutation effects on the 2nd generation after exposure to herbicides. Translated from the French by the Congressional Research Service.
5. Friedman, J. M. Does Agent Orange cause birth defects? *Teratology* **29**:193–221. 1984.
6. Lamb, J. C., J. A. Moore, and T. A. Marks. Evaluation of 2,4-dichlorophenoxyacetic acid (2,4-D) and 2,4,5-trichlorophenoxyacetic acid (2,4,5-T), and 2,3,7,8-tetrachloropdibenzo-*p*-dioxin (TCDD) toxicity in C57BL–6 mice: Reproduction and fertility in treated male mice and evaluation of congenital malformations in their offspring (National Toxicology Program: Research Triangle Park, North Carolina, Publ. NTP-80-44). 1980.
7. Friedman, 1984.[5]
8. Westing, A. H. ed. *Herbicides in War* (Taylor and Francis: London and Philadelphia, 1984).
9. Uhl, M., and T. Ensign. *GI Guinea Pigs* (Wideview Press: New York, 1980). pp. 160-161.
10. Hook, E. B., S. G. Albright, and P. K. Cross. Use of Bernoulli census and long-linear methods for estimating the prevalence of spina bifida in livebirths and the completeness of vital record reports in New York State. *Am. J. Epidemiology* **112**:750–758. 1980.
11. Erickson, J. D., J. Mulinare, P. W. McClain, *et al.* Vietnam veterans' risks for fathering babies with birth defects. *J. Am. Med. Assoc.* **252**:903–912. 1984.
12. Donovan, J. W., R. MacLennan, and M. Adeana. Vietnam service and the risk of congential anomalies: A case–control study. *Medical J. Australia* **140**:394–397. 1984.
13. Friedman, 1984[5]; Dan, B. D. Editorial: Vietnam and birth defects. *J. Am. Med. Assoc.* **252**:936–937. 1984.
14. See Chapter 14.
15. Erickson *et al.*, 1984.[10]

16. Gough, M., and H. Gelband. Review of the Centers for Disease Control's study "Vietnam veterans' risks for fathering babies with health defects." Testimony before Subcommittee on Hospitals and Health Care, Committee on Veterans' Affairs, United States House of Representatives. Oct. 3, 1984.

17. See Fox, J. L. Agent Orange: Guarded reassurance. *Science* **225**:909. 31 Aug. 1984.

18. United States District Court, Eastern District of New York. In re "Agent Orange" product liability litigation. *Loughery v. United States*, No. 81-664, *et al.* Feb. 8, 1985.

19. Donovan *et al.*, 1984.[11]

20. USAF School of Aerospace Medicine. *Project Ranch Hand II: An Epidemiologic Investigation of Health Effects in Air Force Personnel Following Exposure to Herbicides. Baseline Morbidity Results* (Brooks Air Force Base, Texas: United States Air Force, 1984).

21. Hatch, M. Quoted in United States District Court,[18] p. 23. 1985.

22. Stein, Z. Quoted in United States District Court,[18] p. 19. 1985.

23. Nelson, C. J., J. F. Hoson, H. G. Green, *et al.* Retrospective study of the relationship between agricultural use of 2,4,5-T and cleft palate occurrence in Arkansas. *Teratology* **19**:377–384. 1979.

24. Michigan Department of Public Health. Evaluation of congenital malformation rates for Midland and other selected Michigan counties compared nationally and statewide, 1970–1981. Typescript. May 4, 1983.

25. Consultative Council on Congential Abnormalities in the Yarram District. Report. Typescript. Undated.

26. Thomas, H. F. 2,4,5-T use and congenital malformation rates in Hungary. *Lancet*, pp. 214–215. July 26, 1980.

27. See Chapter 9.

28. See, for instance, Shaplen, R. "A Reporter at Large. Return to Vietnam— II." *The New Yorker*, pp. 92 *et seq.* Apr. 29, 1985.

CHAPTER 7

1. This chapter relies heavily on an account pieced together by reporters for the *St. Louis Post-Dispatch*, published in November 14, 1983, the first and most comprehensive such account available.

2. Commoner, B., and R. E. Scott. Accidental contamination of soil with dioxin in Missouri: Effects and Countermeasures. Typescript (St. Louis: Washington University, 1976).

3. Houk, V., Centers for Disease Control. Personal communication, July 1985.

4. Yanders, A., University of Missouri. Personal communication, July 1985.

5. Maskin, A., U.S. Department of Justice. Personal communication, July 1985.

6. Cited in Council on Scientific Affairs. *The Health Effects of "Agent Orange" and Polychlorinated Dioxin Contaminants: An Update, 1984.* Typescript (Chicago: American Medical Association, 1984).

CHAPTER 8

1. *Federal Register*, Vol. 43, No. 78, Friday, April 21, 1978. p. 17,119.
2. *Federal Register*, Vol. 43, No. 78, Friday, April 21, 1978. pp. 17,116–17,144.
3. "The Plowboy Interview: Bonnie Hill." *The Mother Earth News*, No. 72. Nov./Dec. 1981. pp. 17–24.
4. "Report of Assessment of a Field Investigation of Six Year Spontaneous Abortion Rates in Three Oregon Areas in Relation to Forest 2,4,5-T Spray Practices." Environmental Protection Agency. February 28, 1979.
5. *Federal Register*, Vol. 44, No. 52, Thursday, March 15, 1979. pp. 15,874–15,920.
6. Wagner, S. L., Witt, J. M., Norris, L. A., *et al*. A Scientific Critique of the EPA Alsea II Study and Report with the November 16, 1979 Supplement (Cornwallis, Oregon: Oregon State University Environmental Health Sciences Center, October 25, 1979).
7. *Federal Register*, Vol. 44, No. 241, Thursday, December 13, 1979. pp. 72,316–72,341.
8. *Federal Register*, Vol. 48, No. 202, Tuesday, October 18, 1983. pp. 48,434–48,437.
9. Kilpatrick, R. Testimony given in Nunn, 1983,[10] pp. 136–141.
10. Nunn, D. M. Judgment in the Trial between Victoria Palmer et al and Stora Kipparbergs Bergslags Aktiebolag. Supreme Court of Nova Scotia. Sept. 15, 1983.

CHAPTER 9

1. See Chapter 14.
2. See Chapters 10–12.
3. Wipf, H. K, and J. Schmid. Seveso—an environmental assessment. In: *Human and Environmental Risks of Chlorinated Dioxins and Related Compounds*. eds. Tucker, R. E., A. L. Young, and A. P. Gray (New York: Plenum Press, 1983). pp. 255–274.
4. See Chapter 2.
5. See Chapter 8.
6. See Chapter 8.
7. Marni, E., L. Bisanti, L. Abate, *et al*. Birth defects register in Seveso: A TCDD-polluted area. In: *Plans for Clinical and Epidemiologic Follow-up after Area-wide Chemical Contamination* (Washington: National Academy Press, 1982). pp. 174–194.
8. See Chapter 6.
9. Sirchia, G. G., and the Group for Immunological Monitoring. Exposure to TCDD: Immunologic effects. In: *Plans for Clinical and Epidemiologic Follow-up after Area-wide Chemical Contamination* (Washington: National Academy Press, 1982). pp. 234–266.

10. See *Plans for Clinical and Epidemiologic Follow-up after Area-wide Chemical Contamination* (Washington: National Academy Press, 1982).
11. Reggiani, G., Interpharco, Inc., formerly medical director of Roche, Switzerland. Personal communication, July 1985.
12. *Ibid*.
13. See Chapter 7.
14. Yanders, A. F., University of Missouri. Personal communication, July 1985.
15. Wipf and Schmid, 1983.[3]
16. Facchetti, S., A. Balasso, C. Fichtner, *et al*. Studies on the absorption of TCDD by some plant species. Paper presented at American Chemical Society Symposium on Chlorinated Dioxins and Dibenzofurans, Miami, Florida Apr. 29, 1985. See also Dioxins in the environment: No consensus on human hazard. *Chemical and Engineering News*, May 27, 1985. pp. 41–44.
17. Nunn, D. M. Decision in Victoria Palmer et al v. Stora Kopparbergs Bergslags Aktiebolag in the Supreme Court of Nova Scotia. Sept. 15, 1983. p. 175.

CHAPTER 10

1. United States District Court, Southern Court of West Virginia. Durland, J. R. Verbal testimony in James R. Boggess et al versus Monsanto Company. Vol. 7-A. June 26, 1984.
2. United States District Court, Southern Court of West Virginia. Durland, J. R. Verbal testimony in James R. Boggess et al versus Monsanto Company. Vol. 8. June 27, 1984.
3. United States District Court, Southern Court of West Virginia. Kelly, R. E. Verbal testimony in James R. Boggess et al versus Monsanto Company. Vol. 86–A. December 5, 1984. Dr. Kelly was referring to a letter written by Dr. Louis Schwartz on May 11, 1949, that described the white powder.
4. Ashe, W. F., and R. R. Suskind. Reports on chloracne. Monsanto Chemical Company, Nitro, West Virginia. October, 1949 and April, 1950. Typescript. Department of Environmental Health, College of Medicine, University of Cincinnati.
5. Ashe, W. F., and R. R. Suskind. Reports on clinical and environmental surveys from Monsanto Chemical Co., Nitro, West Virginia. 1953. Typescript. Department of Environmental Health, College of Medicine, University of Cincinnati.
6. Durland, 1984.[1]
7. Ashe and Suskind, 1949 and 1950.[4]
8. Ashe and Suskind, 1949 and 1950.[4]
9. Ashe and Suskind, 1953.[5]
10. Moses, M., R. Lilis, K. D. Crow, *et al*. Health status of workers with past exposure to 2,3,7,8-tetrachlorodibenzo-*p*-dioxin in the manufacture of 2,4,5-trichlorophenoxyacetic acid; comparison of findings with and without chloracne. *American J. Industrial Medicine* 5:161–182. 1984.

11. Zack, J. A., and R. R. Suskind. The mortality experience of workers exposed to tetrachlorodibenzodioxin in a trichlorophenol process accident. *J. Occupational Medicine* **22:**11–14. 1980.
12. Zack, J. A., and W. R. Gaffey. A mortality study of workers employed at the Monsanto Company plant in Nitro, West Virginia. In: *Human and Environmental Risks of Chlorinated Dioxins and Related Compounds.* eds. Tucker, R. E., A. L. Young, and A. P. Gray (New York: Plenum Press, 1983). pp. 575–591.
13. Suskind, R. R., and V. S. Hertzberg. Human health effects of 2,4,5-T and its toxic contaminants. *J. American Medical Association* **251:**2372–2380. 1984.
14. Moses *et al.*, 1984.[10]
15. Suskind, R. R., University of Cincinnati. Personal communication, August 1985.

CHAPTER 11

1. See Moses, M., R. Lilis, K. D. Crow, *et al.* Health status of workers with past exposure to 2,3,7,8-tetrachlorodibenzo-*p*-dioxin in the manufacture of 2,4,5-trichlorophenoxyacetic acid; comparison of findings with and without chloracne. *American J. Industrial Medicine* **5:**161–182. 1984.
2. May, G. TCDD: A study of subjects 10 and 14 years after exposure. *Chemosphere* **12:**771–778. 1983.
3. Zack, J. A., and R. R. Suskind. The mortality experience of workers exposed to tetrachlorodibenzodioxin in a trichlorophenol process accident. *J. Occupational Med.* **22:**11–14. 1980; Zack, J. A., and W. R. Gaffey. A mortality study of workers employed at the Monsanto Company plant in Nitro, West Virginia. In: *Human and Environmental Risks of Chlorinated Dioxins and Related Compounds.* eds. Tucker, R. E., A. L. Young, and A. P. Gray (New York: Plenum Press, 1983). pp. 575–591.
4. Thiess, A. M., R. Frentzel-Beyme, and R. Link. Mortality study of persons exposed to dioxin in a trichlorophenol process accident that occurred in the BASF AG on November 17, 1953. *Am. J. Ind. Med.* **3:**179–189. 1982.
5. Dalderup, L. M., and D. Zellenrath. Dioxin exposure: 20 year followup. *Lancet* **1:**1134–1135. Nov. 12, 1983.
6. Bennett, G. The politics of dioxin. *New Scientist,* Jan. 17, 1985. pp. 33–34.
7. May, G. TCDD: 1983.[2]
8. May, G. Chloracne from the accidental production of tetrachlorodibenzodioxin. *British J. Industrial Medicine* **30:**276–283. 1973.
9. May, G. Tetrachlorodibenzodioxin: A survey of subjects ten years after exposure. *British J. Industrial Medicine* **39:**128–135. 1982.
10. Hay, A. *The Chemical Scythe* (New York: Plenum Press, 1982). pp. 109–121.
11. Sell, K. W., 1983. Quoted in Council on Scientific Affairs, American Medical Association. *The Health Effect of "Agent Orange" and Polychlorinated Dioxin Contaminant: An Update. 1984.* Typescript (Chicago: American Medical Association, 1984).
12. Martin, J. The Coalite study. Typescript, 5 pp. and attachments. Undated.

13. Walker, A. E., and J. V. Martin. Lipid profiles in dioxin-exposed workers. *Lancet* **1**:447. Feb. 24, 1979; Martin, J. V. Lipid abnormalities in workers exposed to dioxin. *Brit. J. Ind. Med.* **41**:254–256. 1984.
14. Hay, 1982.[10]
15. *Ibid.*
16. Hobson, L. B. Veterans Administration. Porphyria cutanea tarda. Typescript. 9 pp. April 1983.
17. Bleiberg, J., M. Wallen, R. Brodkin, and I. L. Applebaum. Industrially acquired porphyria. *Archives of Dermatology* **89**:793-797.
18. Poland, A. P., D. Smith, G. Metter, *et al.* A health survey of workers in a 2,4-D and 2,4,5-T plant with special attention to chloracne, porphyria cutanea tarda, and psychologic parameters. *Archives Environmental Health* **22**:316–327. 1971.
19. Pazderova-Vejlupkova, J., M. Nemcova, J. Pickova, *et al.* The development and prognosis of chronic intoxication by tetrachlorodibenzo-*p*-dioxin in men. *Archives Environmental Health* **36**:5–11. 1981.

CHAPTER 12

1. Office of Technology Assessment. *Preventing Illness and Injury in the Workplace* (Washington: Government Printing Office, 1985).
2. Cook, R. R., J. C. Townsend, M. G. Ott, *et al.* Mortality experience of employees exposed to 2,3,7,8-tetrachlorodibenzo-*p*-dioxin (TCDD). *J. Occupational Med.* **22**:530–532. 1980.
3. Ott, M. G., B. B. Holder, and B. S. Olson. A mortality analysis of employees engaged in the manufacture of 2,4,5-trichlorophenoxyacetic acid. *J. Occupational Med.* **22**:47–50. 1980.
4. Young, A. L. Paper presented at the Toxicology Forum, Aspen, Colorado. July 19, 1984.
5. See Chapter 2.
6. Rowe, V. K. Direct testimony (Exhibit 865) in re: The Dow Chemical Company, et al. FIFRA Docket Nos. 415, et al. United States Environmental Protection Agency. Oct. 30, 1980.
7. Davido, F. L. Participant identification interviews: Holmesburg Prison dioxin testing. Typescript, 4 pp. and 3 tables. Obtained from the United States Environmental Protection Agency.
8. Agent Orange papers: What companies knew. *Chemical Week*, July 13, 1983. pp. 24–25; Dioxin: To tell or not to tell. *Chemical Week*, July 13, 1983. p. 3.
9. "7 at Monsanto Lose a Lawsuit over Dioxin Ills." *New York Times.* May 1, 1985. p. 2.
10. See Chapter 10.
11. *New York Times,* May 1, 1985. p. 2.
12. *Ibid.*

CHAPTER 13

1. Hardell, L. Relation of soft tissue sarcoma, malignant lymphoma and colon cancer to phenoxy acids, chlorophenols and other agents. *Scandinavian J. Work Environmental Health* **7**:119–130. 1981; Hardell, L., M. Eriksson, P. Lenner, *et al.* Malignant lymphoma and exposure to chemicals, especially organic solvents, chlorophenols and phenoxy acids: A case–control study. *British J. Cancer* **43**:169–176. 1981.

2. Hardell, L., B. Johansson, and O. Axelson. Epidemiological study of nasal and nasopharyngeal cancer and their relation to phenoxy acid or chlorophenol exposure. *British J. Industrial Medicine* **3**:247–257. 1982.

3. Axelson, O., L. Sundell, K. Andersson, *et al.* An updated epidemiologic investigation on Swedish railroad workers. *Scandinavian J. Work Environmental Health* **6**:73–79. 1980.

4. Hardell, L., and A. Sandstrom. Case control study: Soft tissue sarcomas and exposure to phenoxyacetic acids and chlorophenols. *British J. Cancer* **39**:711–717. 1979; Eriksson, M., L. Hardell, N. O. Berg, *et al.* Soft tissue sarcomas and exposure to chemical substances: A case–referent study. *British J. Industrial Med.* **38**:27–33. 1981; Hardell, L., and M. Eriksson. Soft tissue sarcomas, phenoxy herbicides, and chlorinated phenols. *Lancet* **2**:250. 1981.

5. Hajdu, S. I. Classification and pathological diagnosis of soft tissue sarcomas. In: *Public Health Risks of the Dioxins.* ed. Lowrance, W. W. (William Kaufman: Los Altos, California, 1984). pp. 173–186.

6. Percy, C., E. Stanek, and L. Gloeckler. Accuracy of cancer death certificates and its effect on cancer mortality statistics. *American J. Public Health* **71**:242–250. 1981. Cited in Council on Scientific Affairs. *The Health Effects of "Agent Orange" and Polychlorinated Dioxin Contaminants: An Update, 1984.* Typescript (Chicago: American Medical Association, 1984).

7. Hardell, L., N. O. Bengtsson, U. Jonsson, *et al.* Aetiological aspects on primary liver cancer with special regard to alcohol, organic solvents and acute intermittent porphyria—an epidemiological investigation. *British J. Cancer* **50**:389–397. 1984.

8. Cook, R. R., J. C. Townsend, M. G. Ott, *et al.* Mortality experience of employees exposed to 2,3,7,8-tetrachlorodibenzo-p-dioxin (TCDD). *J. Occupational Med.* **22**:530–532. 1980; Ott, M. G., B. B. Holder, and B. S. Olson. A mortality analysis of employees engaged in the manufacture of 2,4,5-trichlorophenoxyacetic acid. *J. Occupational Med.* **22**:47–50. 1980; Zack, J. A., and R. R. Suskind. The mortality experience of workers exposed to tetrachlorodibenzodioxin in a trichlorophenol process accident. *J. Occupational Med.* **22**:11–14. 1980; Zack, J. A., and W. R. Gaffey. A mortality study of workers employed at the Monsanto Company plant in Nitro, West Virginia. In: *Human and Environmental Risks of Chlorinated Dioxins and Related Compounds.* eds Tucker, R. E., A. L. Young, and A. P. Gray (Plenum Press: New York. 1983). pp. 575–591.

9. Hardell, L., and O. Axelson. Phenoxyherbicides and other pesticides in the

etiology of cancer: Some comments on the Swedish experience. Paper presented at the University of California, San Francisco, December 7–8, 1984.

10. Eklund, G. Does occupational exposure to chemical pesticides increase the cancer risk? *Weed and Plant Protection Conferences.* (Swedish University of Agricultural Sciences Research Information Center: Uppsala. 1983). pp. 6–12. (Translated from the Swedish.)

11. Riihimaki, V., S. Asp, and S. Hernberg. Mortality of 2,4-dichlorophenoxyacetic acid and 2,4,5-trichlorophenoxyacetic acid herbicide applicators in Finland. First report on an ongoing prospective study. *Scandanavian J. Work Environmental Health* **8**:37–42. 1982.

12. Smith, A. H., D. O. Fisher, H. J. Giles, *et al.* The New Zealand soft tissue sarcoma case–control study: Interview findings concerning phenoxyacetic acid exposure. *Chemosphere* **12**:565–571. 1983.

13. See Chapter 4.

14. Cook, R. R. Soft tissue sarcomas: Clues and caution. In: *Human and Environmental Risks of Chlorinated Dioxins and Related Compounds.* eds. Tucker, R. E., A. L. Young, and A. P. Gray (New York: Plenum Press, 1983). pp. 613–618.

15. Hajdu, 1984.[5]

16. Honchar, P. A. and W. E. Halperin. 2,4,5-trichlorophenol and soft tissue sarcoma. *Lancet* **1**:268–269. 1981.

17. Office of Technology Assessment. *Preventing Illness and Injury in the Workplace.* (Washington: Government Printing Office, 1985).

18. Hajdu, 1984.[5]

19. Smith, A. H., N. E. Pearce, D. O. Fisher, *et al.* Soft tissue sarcoma and exposure to phenoxyherbicides and chlorophenols in New Zealand. *J. Natl. Cancer Institute* **73**:1111–1117. 1984.

20. Reference to studies in Hardell and Axelson, 1984.[9]

21. Hardell and Axelson, 1984.[9]

22. See Chapter 12.

23. See the Appendix.

24. Hardell and Axelson, 1984.[9]

CHAPTER 14

1. Doll, R., and R. Peto. The causes of cancer: Quantitative estimates of avoidable risks of cancer in the United States today. *J. Natl. Cancer Institute* **66**:1191–1308. 1981; see also Office of Technology Assessment. *Technologies for Determining Cancer Risks from the Environment* (Government Printing Office: Washington, 1981). Reprinted as *Cancer Risk: Assessing and Reducing the Risks in our Society* (Westview Press: Boulder, Colorado, 1982).

2. Office of Technology Assessment. Smoking-related deaths and financial costs. Typescript. September 1985.

3. Neal, R. A. Biological effects of 2,3,7,8-tetrachlorodibenzo-*p*-dioxin in experimental animals. In: *Public Health Risks of the Dioxins.* ed. Lowrance, W. W. (Los Altos, California: William Kaufman, 1984). pp. 15–29.

4. Peterson, R. E., C. L. Potter, and R. W. Moore. The wasting syndrome and hormonal alterations in 2,3,7,8-tetrachlorodibenzo-p-dioxin toxicity. In: *Public Health Risks of the Dioxins*. ed. Lowrance, W. W. (Los Altos, California: William Kaufman, 1984). pp. 315–350.

5. See Chapter 11 and Dean, J. H., and L. D. Lauer. Immunological effects following exposure to 2,3,7,8-tetrachlorodibenzo-p-dioxin: A review. In: *Public Health Risks of the Dioxins*. ed. Lowrance, W. W. (Los Altos, California: William Kaufman, 1984). pp. 275–294.

6. Lathrop, G., Science Applications International Corporation (formerly principal investigator on the Ranch Hand study before retiring from the Air Force). Personal communication, July 1985.

7. Reggiani, G. Acute human exposure to TCDD in Seveso, Italy. *J. Toxicology Environmental Health* **6**:27–43. 1980.

8. Poland, A., and J. C. Knutson. 2,3,7,8-Tetrachlorodibenzo-p-dioxin and related halogenated aromatic hydrocarbons: Examination of the mechanism of toxicity. *Annual Review Pharmacology Toxicology* **22**:517–554. 1982.

9. Poland, A. P., D. Smith, G. Metter, *et al.* A health survey of workers in a 2,4-D and 2,4,5-T plant. *Archives Environmental Health* **22**:316–327; see also Chapter 11.

10. Poland and Knutson, 1982[8]; Poland, A., J. Knutson, and E. Glover. A consideration of the mechanism of actions of 2,3,7,8-tetrachlorodibenzo-p-dioxin and related halogenated aromatic hydrocarbons. In: *Human and Environmental Risks of Chlorinated Dioxins and Related Compounds*. eds. Tucker, R. E., A. L. Young, and A. P. Gray (New York: Plenum Press, 1983). pp. 539–559.

11. Ames, B. N. Dietary carcinogens and anti-carcinogens. *Sciences* **221**:1256–1264. 1983.

12. See Marx, J. L. The cytochrome P450's and their genes. *Science* **228**:975–976. 1985.

13. Neal, 1984.[3]

14. Mortelmans, K., S. Haworth, W. Speck, *et al.* Mutagenicity testing of Agent Orange components and related chemicals. *Toxicology Applied Pharmacology* **75**:137–146. 1984; E. Zeiger, NTP. Private communication, December 1984.

15. Poland, A., and E. Glover. An estimate of the maximum *in vivo* covalent binding of 2,3,7,8-tetrachlorodibenzo-p-dioxin to rat liver protein, ribosomal RNA, and DNA. *Cancer Research* **39**:3341–3344. 1979.

16. National Toxicology Program. *Carcinogenesis Bioassay of 2,3,7,8-tetrachlorodibenzo-p-dioxin in Swiss-Webster Mice (Dermal Study)* (National Institutes of Health: Washington, 1982).

17. Kociba, R. J. Summary and critique of rodent carcinogenicity studies of chlorinated bibenzo-p-dioxins. In: *Public Health Risks of the Dioxins*. ed. Lowrance, W. W. (Los Altos, California: William Kaufman, 1984). pp. 77–98.

18. National Toxicology Program. *Carcinogenesis Bioassay of 2,3,7,8-tetrachlorodibenzo-p-dioxin in Osborne-Mendel rats and B6C3F1 Mice (Gavage Study)*. (National Institutes of Health: Washington, 1982).

19. Kociba, R. J., D. G. Keyes, J. E. Beyer, *et al.* Results of a two-year chronic

toxicity and oncogenicity study of 2,3,7,8-tetrachlorodibenzo-*p*-dioxin in rats. *Toxicology and Applied Pharmacology* **46**:279–303. 1978.

20. *Public Health Risks of the Dioxins*. ed. W. W. Lowrance (Los Altos, California: William Kaufman, 1984).

21. Rozman, J. Q., T. Rozman, and H. Greim. Effect of thyroidectomy and thyroxine on 2,3,7,8-tetrachlorodibenzo-*p*-dioxin (TCDD) induced toxicity. *Toxicology Applied Pharmacology* **72**:372–376. 1984; cited in Council on Scientific Affairs. *The Health Effects of "Agent Orange" and Polychlorinated Dioxin Contaminants: An Update, 1984.* Typescript (Chicago: American Medical Association, 1984).

22. Berenblum, I., and P. Shubik. A new quantitative approach to the study of the stages of chemical carcinogenesis in the mouse's skin. *British J. Cancer* **1**:383–391. 1947.

23. Poland, A., D. Palen, and E. Glover. Tumour promotion by TCDD in skin of Hrs/J hairless mice. *Nature* **300**:271–273. 1982.

24. Pitot, H. C., T. Goldsworthy, H. A. Campbell, and A. Poland. Quantitative evaluation of the promotion by 2,3,7,8-tetrachlorodibenzo-*p*-dioxin of hepatocarcinogenesis from diethylnitrosamine. *Cancer Research* **40**:3616–3620. 1980.

25. Zeise, L., R. Wilson, and E. Crouch. Use of acute toxicity to estimate carcinogenic risk. *Risk Analysis* **4**:187–199. 1984; Zeise, L., E. A. C. Crouch, and R. Wilson. A possible relationship between toxicity and carcinogenicity. Typescript. 1986. Submitted.

26. Aldred, J. E., B. S. Belcher, Christopher, A. J., *et al.* Report of the consultative council on congenital abnormalities in the Yarram district. Presented to the Australian Parliament. Typescript. viii + 55 pp. 1978.

27. McNulty, W. P. Fetocidal and teratogenic actions of TCDD. In: *Public Health Risks of the Dioxins.* ed. Lowrance, W. W. (Los Altos, California: William Kaufman, 1984). pp. 245–253.

28. Rodricks, J. V. Some general observations on the safety of PCDDs. In: *Human and Environmental Risks of Chlorinated Dioxins and Related Compounds.* eds. Tucker, R. E., A. L. Young, and A. P. Gray (New York: Plenum Press, 1983). pp. 629–634; Longstreth, J. D., and J. M. Hushon. Risk assessment for 2,3,7,8-tetrachlorodibenzo-*p*-dioxin (TCDD). In: *Human and Environmental Risks of Chlorinated Dioxins and Related Compounds.* eds. Tucker, R. E., A. L. Young, and A. P. Gray (New York: Plenum Press, 1983). pp. 639–665.

29. Council on Scientific Affairs. *The Health Effects of "Agent Orange" and Polychlorinated Dioxin Contaminants: An Update, 1984.* Typescript (Chicago: American Medical Association, 1984). p. 41.

CHAPTER 15

1. "$4 Million Cleanup of Dioxin Is Starting at Sites in Newark." *New York Times,* Jan. 20, 1985. p. A20.

2. "Dioxin Detected in Barrels on Upstate Golf Course." *New York Times*, Feb. 17, 1985. p. 48.
3. "The Truth about Agent Orange." *New York Times*, Aug. 13, 1984. p. A22; "Orangemail: Why It Got Paid." *New York Times*, Mar. 8, 1985. p. A34.
4. Nunn, D. M. Decision in Victoria Palmer et al v. Stora Kopparbergs Bergslags Aktiebolag in the Supreme Court of Nova Scotia. Sept. 15, 1983. p. 180.
5. Barnes, D. G. U.S. Environmental Protection Agency's *Dioxin Strategy: Executive Summary*. In: *Public Health Risks of the Dioxins*. ed. Lowrance, W. W. (Los Altos, California: William Kaufman, 1984). pp. 373–380.
6. Office of Technology Assessment. *Superfund Strategy*. (Washington: Government Printing Office, 1985).
7. See Chapter 11.
8. See Chapter 6.
9. Ableson, P. H. Chlorinated dioxins [editorial]. *Science* **220**:1337. 1983.
10. Sterling, T. D. Health effects of dioxin [letter]. *Science* **221**:1202. 1984.
11. See Chapter 13.
12. Hay, A., and E. Silbergeld. Assessing the risk of dioxin exposure [letter]. *Nature* **315**:102–103. 1985.
13. Gorman, J. "Tooth and Paw." *The New Yorker*. Dec. 24, 1984. p. 29
14. Greenleaf, S. *Fatal Obsession* (Ballantine Books: New York, 1983).
15. Cussler, C. *Deep Six* (Pocket Books: New York, 1984). pp. 29–30.
16. "U.S. Agency Orders Removal of PCB's." *New York Times*. July 3, 1985. p. A17.
17. Bellin, J. S., and D. Barnes. Health hazard assessment for chlorinated dioxins and -dibenzofurans other than 2,3,7,8-TCDD. Typescript. EPA: Washington. Sept. 26, 1984. And "Draft EPA health document says dibenzofurans may be as deadly as dioxin." *Inside E.P.A.*,5(44):14 November 2, 1984.
18. Barnes, D. Trip report. Lombardy Region Symposium on Dioxin, Milan, Italy, Sept. 19–22, 1984. Undated typescript.
19. Hardell, L., L. Domellof, and M. Nygren. Levels of polychlorinated dibenzodioxins and dibenzofurans in adipose tissue of patients with soft-tissue sarcoma or malignant lymphoma exposed to phenoxy acids and of unexposed controls. Submitted to *Scandinavian J. Work Environmental Health*. 1986.

CHAPTER 16

1. Lowrance, W. W. Interpretive summary of the symposium. In: *Public Health Risks of the Dioxins*. ed. Lowrance, W. W. (William Kaufman: Los Altos, California, 1984). pp. 3–14.
2. Scheuplein, R. Proposed Food and Drug Administration approach to tolerance-setting for dioxins in food. In: *Public Health Risks of the Dioxins*. ed. Lowrance, W. W. (William Kaufman: Los Altos, California, 1984). pp. 367–372.

3. Environmental Protection Agency. Ambient water quality criteria for 2,3,7,8-tetrachlorodibenzo-p-dioxin (U.S.E.P.A.: Washington, Feb. 1984).

4. Kimbrough R. D., H. Falk, P. Stehr, et al. Health implications of 2,3,7,8-tetrachlorodibenzo-p-dioxin (TCDD) contamination of residential soil. In: Public Health Risks of the Dioxins. ed. Lowrance, W. W. (William Kaufman: Los Altos, California, 1984a). pp. 121–150; same authors and title. J. Toxicology Environmental Health 14:47–93. 1984b.

5. Kimbrough et al., 1984a, b.[4]

6. Scheuplin, 1984[2]; Food and Drug Administration. FDA advises Great Lakes States to monitor dioxin-contaminated fish. Food Drug Cosmetic Law Reports, paragraph 41, 321. (Commerce Clearing House: Washington, Sept. 8, 1981).

7. EPA, 1984.[3]

8. Moore, J. A. Issues in environmental toxicology and chemical analysis. Paper presented before the Association of Official Analytical Chemists. Oct. 31, 1984.

9. Kociba, R. J., D. G. Keyes, J. E. Beyer, et al. Results of a two-year chronic toxicity and oncogenicity study of 2,3,7,8-tetrachlorodibenzo-p-dioxin in rats. Toxicology and Applied Pharmacology 46:279–303. 1978.

10. EPA, 1984.[3]

11. Young, A. L. Determination and measurement of human exposure to the debenzo-p-dioxins. Bulletin Environmental Contamination Toxicology 33:702–709. 1984; Raloff, J. Dioxin: Is everyone contaminated? Science News 128:26–29. July 13, 1985.

12. Gehring, P. Background exposure to 2,3,7,8-tetrachlorodibenzo-p-dioxin. In: Public Health Risks of the Dioxins. ed. Lowrance, W. W. (William Kaufman: Los Altos, California 1984). pp. 151–154.

13. Gehring, P. J., P. G. Watanabe, and G. E. Blau. Pharmacokinetic studies in evaluation of the toxicological and environmental hazard of chemicals. In: New Concepts in Safety Evaluation (Hemisphere Publishing: Washington, 1976).

14. Stallings, D. L., L. M. Smith, J. D. Petty, et al. Residues of polychlorinated dibenzo-p-dioxins and dibenzofurans in Laurentian Great Lakes fish. In: Human and Environmental Risks of Chlorinated Dioxins and Related Compounds. eds. Tucker, R. E., A. L. Young, and A. P. Gray (Plenum Press: New York, 1983). pp. 221–240.

15. Firestone, D. Paper presented at the national meeting of the American Chemical Society, Miami, Florida. Apr. 29, 1985; Scheuplein, R. FDA. Personal communication, July 1985.

16. Facchetti, S., A. Balasso, C. Fichtner, et al. Studies on the absorption of TCDD by some plant species. Paper presented to the national meeting of the American Chemical Society, Miami, Florida. Apr. 28, 1985.

17. Hardell, L., L. Domellof, and M. Nygren. Levels of polychlorinated dibenzodioxins and dibenzofurans in adipose tissue of patients with soft-tissue sarcoma or malignant lymphoma exposed to phenoxy acids and of unexposed controls. Submitted to Scandinavian J. Work Environmental Health. 1986.

18. Environmental Protection Agency. *Dioxin Strategy* (Washington: EPA, 1983).
19. Environmental Protection Agency. Interim list of tier I and II sites. Typescript. Obtained from the EPA, July 1985.
20. Commoner, B. Environmental and economic analysis of alternative municipal solid waste disposal technologies. I. An assessment of the risks due to emissions of chlorinated dioxins and dibenzofurans from proposed New York City incinerators. City University of New York. May 1, 1984; Wald, M. L. "Dioxin Held Slight in Studies of City Garbage Fuel Project." *New York Times*, Sept. 26, 1984. p. A1.
21. Fred C. Hart Associates, Inc. *Assessment of Potential Public Health Impacts Associated with Predicted Emissions of Polychlorinated Dibenzo-Dioxins and Polychlorinated Dibenzo-Furans from the Brooklyn Navy Yard Resource Recovery Facility.* Aug. 17, 1984.
22. Konheim and Ketcham and the Environmental Science Laboratory, Mt. Sinai School of Medicine. *Evaluation of the Risk of Dioxins and Furans from the Proposed Brooklyn Navy Yard Resource Recovery Facility.* March 1985.
23. Steisel, N. Letter to the editor. *New York Times*, Jan. 26, 1985.
24. Mathewson, J. "Blue Goose" lives on diet of dioxin. *Science News* **128**:39. July 20, 1985.
25. Smith, R. M., D. R. Hilker, P. W. O'Keefe, *et al.* Determination of tetrachlorodibenzo-*p*-dioxin and tetrachlorodibenzofurans in environmental samples by high performance liquid chromatography, capillary gas chromatography and high resolution mass spectrometry. In: *Human and Environmental Risks of Chlorinated Dioxins and Related Compounds.* eds. Tucker, R. E., A. L. Young, and A. P. Gray (Plenum Press: New York, 1983). pp. 73–94.
26. Council on Scientific Affairs. *The Health Effects of "Agent Orange" and Polychlorinated Dioxin Contaminants: An Update, 1984.* Typescript (Chicago: American Medical Association, 1984).
27. See *Public Health Risks of the Dioxins.* ed. Lowrance, W. W. (William Kaufman: Los Altos, California, 1984); Council on Scientific Affairs,1984.[26]
28. Ames, B. N., and A. H. Rosenfeld. Letter to Representatives J. Scheurer, C. Schneider, and Don Ritter. June 3, 1985.
29. Wilson, R., Harvard University. Personal communication, July 1985.

APPENDIX

1. Calculation of the amount of dioxin that reached the ground from Operation Ranch Hand spray missions. No allowance is made for drift away from the target or inactivation of dioxin.

   The rate of application of Agent Orange was 3 gallons per acre:

   3 gals/acre $\times$ 3.785 liters/gal = 11.4 liters/acre (conversion of gals/acre to liters/acre)

   11.4 liters/acre $\times$ acre/4047 m^2 = 11.4 liters/4047 m^2 (conversion of liters/acre to liters/m^2)

   11.4 liters/4047 m^2 = 0.0028 liter/m^2 = 2.8 ml m^2 (conversion of liters/m^2 to milliliters/m^2)

2.8 ml/m^2 × 1.28 g/ml = 3.6 g/m^2 (correction for density of Agent Orange)
3.6 g/m^2 × 50 × 10^{-6} = 180 × 10^{-6} g/m^2 = 180 microg/m^2 (fraction of Agent Orange that was dioxin)
180 microg/m^2 × 0.18 m^2/(area of man's head and shoulders) = 32.4 microg/man

Young et al., 1978,[2] reported that no more than 6% of the total spray would reach the ground under a jungle canopy.

2. Young, A. L., J. A. Calcagni, C. E. Thalken, et al. The Toxicology, Environmental Fate, and Human Risk of Herbicide Orange and Its Associated Dioxin (Brooks Air Force Base, Texas: USAF Occupational and Environmental Health Laboratory, 1978). p. 1–23.

3. See Chapter 2.

4. Rowe, V. K., Dow Chemical Company. Direct testimony before the Environmental Protection Agency. FIFRA Docket Nos. 415, et al. Date served: October 30, 1980.

5. Scheuplein, R. Proposed Food and Drug Administration approach to tolerance-setting for dioxins in food. In: Public Health Risks of the Dioxins, ed. Lowrance, W. W. (Los Altos, California: William Kaufman, 1984). pp. 367–372.

6. Stevens, K. M. Agent Orange toxicity: A quantitative perspective. Human Toxicology 1:31–39. 1981.

7. Centers for Disease Control, Agent Orange Projects Office. Exposure assessment for the Agent Orange Study. Interim report number 2. Supplemental information. Typescript. December 8, 1985.

INDEX

AAAS. *See* American Association for the Advancement of Science (AAAS)
Acceptable level, 16
  See also Exposure level
Administrative law, 228
  See also Lawsuits
Agent Blue, 60
Agent Orange
  birth defects and, 56, 105–120
  cancer and, 46, 64
  causation and, 89
  compensation and, 224
  Congress (U.S.) and, 63–64
  corporate response and, 184
  dioxin content of, 19, 34
  dioxin exposure and, 35–36, 259–262
  effectiveness of, 52–54
  epidemiology and, 61
  future impact of, 89–104
  ground troops and, 59–60, 76–79
  law and, 25–26
  lawsuits and, 84–87, 221–222
  politics and, 56–57
  quantities of, 51
  Ranch Hand study and, 68–76
  studies and, 229–230, 231–232
  Veterans Administration and, 46–47
  veteran's health and, 63–87

Agent Orange (*cont.*)
  Vietnam War and, 8, 43–61
  See also Dioxin
Agent Orange Working Group, 91–92, 93, 94–95, 254
Alcoholics, 179
Alsea studies, 140, 143, 201–219
American Association for the Advancement of Science (AAAS), 55, 57
American Medical Association (AMA), 218, 253–254
Animal studies, 201–219
  birth defects and, 105, 106
  cancer and, 194, 203–207, 212–213
  causation and, 208–210
  chloracne and, 30, 187
  dioxin studies and, 22, 213–231
  government and, 238
  liver cancer and, 194–195
  risk and, 218–219
  2, 4, 5–T and, 138, 139
  validity of, 107, 202–203, 205
  See also Studies and study design
Asbestos, 27, 181
Australia, 76–78, 110

BASF plant (Germany), 174
Bhopal, India, 149
Biological warfare, *See* Chemical and biological warfare

281

Birth defects
  Agent Orange and, 56, 105–120
  animal tests and, 214–216
  Centers for Disease Control
      study, 255–256
  compensation and, 225
  dioxin and, 19, 20, 47, 118
  government policy and, 115
  Nitro studies and, 170
  Seveso accident and, 152–153
  Vietnam, 59
  See also Miscarriages
Bladder cancer, 164–165
  See also Cancer
Bliss, Russell M., 123, 124–125, 128,
      134–135
Boy Scouts of America, 13–15, 18
Bricker, Jerome, 93
Bunker, Ellsworth, 55
Burford, Anne, 133, 134, 232

Cancer
  Agent Orange and, 46, 64
  animal tests and, 203–207, 212–
      213, 238
  body fat dioxin levels and, 244
  causation and, 67, 205–206
  Centers for Disease Control
      study and, 99
  chemical carcinogens, 47
  cigarette smoking and, 147–148
  death rates and, 66–67
  diet and, 206
  dioxin exposure and, 15, 19, 20,
      173–174, 193–200
  dose–response concept and, 181
  epidemiology and, 67–68
  exposure levels and, 251
  infantry study and, 77
  NIOSH and, 229
  Nitro studies and, 165, 168–169
  p-aminobiphenyl and, 164–165
  Ranch Hand study and, 73, 81
  registry concept and, 175

Cancer (cont.)
  soft tissue sarcomas, 78–79, 193–
      200
  study design and, 21
  See also entries under names of spe-
      cific cancers
Carcinogens, 67, 203–207
Carter, Coleman, 127
Case-control studies, 195–196
Causation
  Agent Orange and, 89
  animal tests and, 208–210
  cancer and, 67, 205–206
  disease and, 66
  environment and, 227
  lawsuits and, 223
  mutations and, 211–212
Centers for Disease Control (CDC)
  acceptable level of dioxin deci-
      sion and, 16, 240–241
  birth defects study, 108, 110,
      111–112, 255–256
  cohort study by, 95–103
  compensation and, 225
  exposure levels and, 151
  safe levels and, 240–241
  soft tissue sarcomas and, 199
  Times Beach and, 126–129, 134
Chemical and biological warfare,
      54–55
Chemical industry
  chloracne and, 29–30
  dioxin exposure and, 34–35, 36,
      37, 99
  self-policing in, 188
  See also Industrial exposure; en-
      tries under names of specific
      companies
Chemical waste. See Waste disposal
Children, 13–15
  See also Birth defects;
      Miscarriages
Chloracne
  chemical industry and, 29–33,
      184, 185, 186

Chloracne (*cont.*)
  dioxin and, 29, 33
  dose–response and, 182
  human experiments, 185–186,
    187–188
  industrial exposure and, 176,
    178–179
  Nitro explosion and, 159–160,
    161–162, 163–164, 167–168
  Seveso accident and, 140, 154
  Times Beach and, 127
  Vietnam veterans and, 80, 94
Chlordane, 27
Chlorinated aromatic hydrocarbons
  29–30
Cigarette smoking
  cancer risk and, 147–148, 205–206
  Ranch Hand study and, 81
Coal fires, 41
Coalite plant (England), 174, 175–
  178
Cohort studies
  cancer and, 195
  Centers for Disease Control and,
    95–103
  Ranch Hand study, 69
Compensation
  Agent Orange and, 64
  lawsuits and, 224–225
Comprehensive Environmental Re-
  sponse, Compensation, and
  Liability Act ("Superfund
  Act"), 135
Congress (U.S.)
  Agent Orange and, 63–64
  compensation and, 225
  studies and, 92
  See also Government
Contamination, defined, 13n
Corporate response, 183–192
  See also Chemical industry; *entries*
    under names of specific
    companies
Costle, Douglas, 143
Court cases. *See* Lawsuits

Cussler, Clive, 233
Cytochrome P-450, 209–210

Danforth, John C., 133
Daschle, Tom, 176
Death certificates, 194
Death rates. *See* Mortality rates
Defoliation, 52–54, 55–56
Department of Defense (DOD). *See*
  United States Department of
  Defense
Diamond Alkali (Diamond
  Shamrock), 179, 188
Diet, 206
Dioxin
  Agent Orange and, 35–36, 43, 92,
    259–262
  animal studies, 22, 201–219
  birth defects and, 47, 105, 118
  cancer and, 193–200
  children and, 13–15
  chloracne and, 33
  corporate response and, 183–192
  creation of, 27–28
  dose-response concept and, 181
  environmental presence of, 36–
    37, 239–246
  exposure levels and, 60, 181,
    240–242
  exposure to, 8
  fires and, 38–40, 248
  heart disease and, 182
  herbicides and, 33–34
  hexachlorophene and, 122
  immune system and, 209
  industrial exposure to, 173–182
  lawsuits and, 221–235
  media and, 221
  mutagens and, 113
  Nitro studies and, 170
  risks and, 7, 228
  Seveso (Italy) and, 149–156
  Times Beach and, 121–136
    toxicity of, 19–20, 21, 37–38,
    225–226

Dioxin (*cont.*)
  2,4,5-T and, 138
  ubiquitousness of, 7, 245
  Vietnam War and, 8
  See also Agent Orange; *entries under names of dioxin-containing chemicals*
Disease
  causation and, 66
  See also Cancer; *entries under names of specific diseases*
DNA, 209, 210–213
Doll, Richard, 205, 206
Dose–response concept, 181
  See also Exposure level
Dow Chemical Company, 28, 38
  attacks on, 227–228
  chloracne and, 184–185, 186
  corporate response and, 184
  monitoring methods, 188
  suit against, 84–85
  2,4,5-T and, 138, 140, 145–147, 237

Eagleton, Thomas, 133
EDB, 27
Educational achievement, 166–167
Ensign, Tod, 107
Environment, 227
Environmental Defense Fund, 227
Environmental Protection Agency (EPA), 14
  environmental hazards and, 208, 245–246
  exposure levels and, 239–241
  Fort A. P. Hill and, 16–18
  resources of, 20
  still bottom disposal and, 36–37
  Times Beach and, 130–131, 134
  2,4,5-T and, 138–141, 143–146, 237
Environment Canada, 39
Enzymes, 209–211

Epidemiology
  administrative law and, 228
  Agent Orange and, 61
  cancer and, 67–68
  Centers for Disease Control study, 95
  developing countries and, 230
  difficulties in, 22
  exposure level and, 181
  Ranch Hand study and, 68–76
  risk and, 23–24, 223
  sex differences and, 250–251
  study design and, 140–141
  See also Studies and study design
Esteron 3-3E, 147
Expert witnesses, 222
Exposure levels, 93–94
  animal tests and, 214
  birth defects and, 113, 215–216
  body fat accumulation and, 242–244
  chloracne and, 140
  corporate response and, 184–185
  epidemiology and, 181
  lawsuits and, 222–223
  Seveso plant and, 151
  statistics of, 240–242
  study design and, 113–114
  2,4,5-T study and, 142–143
  Vietnam war and, 98–99

Federal Insecticide, Fungicide, and Rodenticide Act (FIFRA), 137, 138
Federal Resource Conservation and Recovery Act, 135
Feinberg, Kenneth, 84
Fires
  dioxin production and, 28, 38–40, 238–239
  furans and, 234–235
  future and, 246–247
  See also Incineration
Fish, 239–240, 243, 245–246

Food and Drug Administration
  animal studies and, 238
  saccharin and, 203
Food chain, 239–240, 243, 244–246
Ford, Gerald, 58
Fort A. P. Hill, 13–15
  aceptable levels and, 20
  EPA and, 16–18
Furans, 234, 235

Gelband, Hellen, 9, 113
General Accounting Office (GAO),
      90, 91
Gorsuch, Anne. See Burford, Anne
Government
  animal testing and, 204, 238
  birth defects and, 115
  carcinogens and, 205
  distrust of, 16, 255
  environmental hazards and, 207–
      208
  Fort A. P. Hill and, 18–19
  infantry men and, 89–90, 91–92
  Ranch Hand study and, 83–84
  research expenditures of, 26
  science and, 24–25
  Times Beach and, 130, 133, 134
Ground water. See Water supply

Hampel, Frank, 125, 128
Hansen, John, 90
Harris, Daniel J., 130
Hart, Philip, 56
Hay, Alastair, 178
Heart disease
  dioxin and, 173–174, 182
  Nitro studies and, 163, 165, 168–
      169, 171
  Ranch Hand study and, 81
Herbicide Assessment Committee
      (HAC), 57
Herbicide Orange, 52
  See also Agent Orange
Herbicides
  dioxin content in, 33–34

Herbicides (cont.)
  toxicity of, 19
  2,4,5-T, 137–148
  U.S. military use of, 60–61
  U.S. policy and, 58–59
  Vietnam war and, 49–51
  See also 2,4,5-T (herbicide)
Hercules Incorporated, 138
Hexachlorophene, 122
Hill, Bonnie, 139–140, 141, 143, 144
Hoffman-Taff Company, 122
Human studies
  difficulties in, 21–22, 23
  See also Animal studies; Epi-
        demiology; Studies and
        . study design
Hyde Park Dump (New York), 37
Hydrocarbons, 29–30

Immune system, 209
Impotence, 169–170
Incineration
  dioxin disposal, 36, 246–249
  dioxin production, 246–248
  See also Fires
Industrial exposure, 173–182
Infantrymen
  government and, 89–90
  study of, 76–79

Kimbrough, Renate, 133
Kinman, Riley, 124

Latent period, 67
Lavelle, Rita, 133, 134
Lawsuits
  administrative law, 228
  Agent Orange and, 84–87
  awards in, 25–26
  birth defects and, 117–118
  causation and, 223
  compensation and, 224–225
  corporate response and, 190–191
  dioxin and, 221–235
  exposure levels and, 222–223

Lawsuits (*cont.*)
  media and, 226
  Nitro case and, 191
  Nova Scotia case 147–148, 221
  Time Beach and, 135
Lee, John W., 122, 123
Libido, 169–170
Lindane, 27
Liver
  animal studies and, 194–195, 214
  dioxin and, 154
  industrial exposure and, 178–179
  Nitro explosion and, 160, 162
  Ranch Hand study and, 80
Love Canal, 37
Lowrance, William, 237–238

Mangroves, 55–56, 58
Martin, Jennifer, 177, 178
May, George, 176, 177
McCarthy, Frank, 46
Media
  Agent Orange and, 87
  dioxin and, 7
  dioxin toxicity and, 221
  lawsuits and, 226
  perceived threat and, 16
  Ranch Hand study and, 83
Medical care, 183–184
Meselson, Matthew, 57
Methyl isocyanate gas, 149
Metropolitan Atlanta Congenital
    Birth Defects Program, 108
Michaels, Edwin, 122, 123
Minker, Harold, 129
Miscarriages
  dioxin and, 19, 20, 106
  exposure level and, 251
  study design and, 141–142
  2,4,5-T and, 139–140, 141
  Vietnam and, 59
  See also Birth defects
Missouri. *See* Times Beach
    (Missouri)

Monsanto Company, 157, 159, 160,
    161, 162, 164, 166, 183, 188,
    190–191
Moore, John 241
Morrison, S. E., 47
Mortality rates
  Australian study, 76–78
  cancer and, 66–67
  Centers for Disease Control and,
    97
  dioxin and, 182
  Nitro studies and, 163, 164, 165–
    166
  Ranch Hand study and, 70, 71,
    72–76
  studies and, 230–231
Moses, Marion, 166, 169
Mutation
  causation and, 211–212
  dioxin and, 113, 210–211
  radiation and, 211

National Academy of Sciences
    (NAS)
  Agent Orange and, 57–58
  Ranch Hand study and, 69
National Cancer Institute, 194
  animal testing and, 204
  soft tissue sarcomas and, 199–200
National Institute for Occupational
    Safety and Health (NIOSH)
  exposure levels and, 253
  registry, 175
  soft tissue sarcomas and, 197–
    198, 229
National Institutes of Health (NIH)
  animal testing and, 204
  Nitro studies and, 166
National Toxicology Program, 204–
    205
Nerve damage
  emphasis on, 252–253
  Nitro explosion, 160, 162, 169
New York City, 246–248

Nitro (West Virginia) explosion,
    157–171
  corporate response and, 183
  decontamination efforts, 173
  lawsuits, 191
Nixon, Richard M., 56
Northeastern Pharmaceutical and
    Chemical Company, 122

Occupational medicine
  advances in, 184
  specialty of, 183
Office of Technology Assessment
    (OTA), 10, 205–206, 254
Operation Ranch Hand, 49–51
  ground troops and, 59–60
  politics and, 54
  See also Agent Orange; Ranch
    Hand studies; Vietnam war
Orians, Gordon H., 56

p-aminobiphenyl, 164–165
PCBs. See Polychlorinated bi-
    phenyls (PCBs)
Percy, Charles, 90
Pesticides
  dioxin exposure and, 35
  Environmental Protection Agency
    and, 138
  See also Herbicides
Peto, Richard, 205, 206
Pfeiffer, E. W., 56
Phillips, J., 128–129
Phillips-Duphar plant (Holland),
    174
Piatt, Andrea, 125, 126
Piatt, Judy, 125, 128
Plastics fires, 40
Poland, Alan, 209, 214
Politics
  Agent Orange and, 56–57
  Operation Ranch Hand and, 54
  science and, 54–55
  See also Government

Polychlorinated biphenyls (PCBs),
    234, 249
Porphyria cutanea tarda
  compensation and, 224
  industrial exposure and, 178–179,
    180
Psychological factors
  industrial exposure and, 180–181
  Nitro studies and, 167–168, 170–
    171
  Ranch Hand study and, 80–83

Radiation, 211
Radon gas, 256
Ranch Hand studies, 68–76
  birth defects and, 115, 116–117
  dioxin exposure calculations,
    259–262
  infantrymen and, 90
  policy making and, 83–84
  subjective factors and, 80–83
  See also Agent Orange; Operation
    Ranch Hand; Vietnam war
Reagan, Ronald, 26, 52, 133, 180,
    207
Registry, 175
Reutershan, Paul, 46, 66, 67, 68, 84
Risk
  animal studies and, 218–219
  difficulties of, 23–24
Roche Pharmaceuticals, 151
Rumack, Barry H., 14, 16

Saccharin, 203
Sandermann, W., 31, 33
Schulz, Karl, 29, 30, 31, 33, 163,
    185–186
Science
  government and, 24–25
  politics and, 54–55
  See also Animal studies,
    Epidemiology
Seveso (Italy), 149–156, 178
Sex differences, 250–251

Silvex, 138n. *See also* 2,4,5-
    Trichlorophenol
Skin disease
    dioxin and, 29
    industrial exposure and, 178–179,
        180
    See also Chloracne; Porphyria cut-
        anea tarda
Soft tissue sarcomas, 78–79, 193–
        200
    Centers for Disease Control
        study and, 99
    classification of, 194
    NIOSH and, 229
    Ranch Hand studies and, 81
    studies and, 196–200
    See also Cancer
Sorge, George, 31, 33
Spina bifida, 107–108
    See also Birth defects
Spontaneous abortion. *See*
        Miscarriages
Stahl, Frank, 57
Statistical significance, 70n
Stillbirths. *See* Miscarriages
Still bottoms, 36–37, 123
Stomach cancer, 174
    See also Cancer
Stout, Vernon, 129
Studies and study design
    cancer and, 195–196, 199
    costs of, 65
    imperfections in, 118–119
    Nitro population, 163–171
    2,4,5-T and, 140–141, 144–145
    See also Animal studies; Epi-
        demiology; *entries under
        names of specific studies*
Sunlight, 37
Superfund, 135–136
Suskind, R., 163, 166, 169
Syntex Corporation, 128–129, 130

Testicular cancer, 67–68
    See also Cancer

Thomas, Lee, 133, 134
Thymus gland
    animal tests, 208
    dioxin and, 153
Times Beach (Missouri), 121–136
    dioxin contamination in, 37
    safe levels and, 240–241
Toxic Substances Control Act, 208
Trichlorophenol
    dioxin and, 224
    dioxin exposure and, 34
    dioxin production and, 28
    herbicides and, 138–139
    production workers and, 183–184
    Times Beach and, 122
Tschirley, Fred S., 55, 56
2,3,7,8-tetrachlorobenzene-*p*-dioxin,
        15–16n
2,4,5-Trichlorophenol, 16n, 137–148
    dioxin content of, 138, 146–147,
        189
    Dow Chemical and, 237
    miscarriages and, 143–144
    regulation of, 137–140, 143, 145–
        147, 138
    study design and, 144–145
    uses of, 137–138

Uhl, Michael, 107
Ulcers, 168
United States Department of
        Agriculture
    dioxin and, 56
    2,4,5-T and, 137, 138
United States Department of
        Defense
    Agent Orange and, 56, 68
    infantrymen and, 89, 90
    Vietnam war and, 55
United States Public Health Service,
        183

Veterans Administration
    Agent Orange and, 46–47
    cohort study and, 95

Veterans Administration (*cont.*)
  medical treatment and, 26
  skin diseases and, 180
  Vietnam experience study, 93
Vietnam Experience study, 95–103
Vietnam Memorial, 44–45
Vietnam war
  birth defects and, 109, 110
  defoliation and, 52–54
  dioxin and, 8, 35–36
  disease and, 45–46
  ecology and, 55–56
  herbicides and, 49–51
  military tactics and, 47, 48–49, 54
  public opinion and, 43–45
  See also Operation Ranch Hand;
    Ranch Hand studies

Waste disposal
  dioxin exposure and, 36
  dioxin production and, 246–248
  risks and, 224
Water and Wastewater Technical
    School, 124
Water supply
  dioxin levels and, 239
  Times Beach and, 123–124
Weinstein, Jack B., 84, 85, 115
Wilcox, F. A., 46, 54, 67
Wind dispersion, 40
Wood fires. *See* Fires

Yannacone, Victor, 46, 84

Zack, Judith, 163
Zack, Matthew, 127